Comprehensive Management of Spina Bifida

Editor

Harold L. Rekate, M.D.
Chief, Pediatric Neurosurgery
Barrow Neurological Institute
Phoenix, Arizona

CRC Press
Boca Raton   Ann Arbor   Boston

CP 23681 (10)

Library of Congress Cataloging-in-Publication Data

Comprehensive management of spina bifida / editor, Harold L. Rekate.
   p.   cm.
   Includes bibliographies and index.
   ISBN 0-8493-0151-3
   1. Myelomeningocele—Treatment. I. Rekate, Harold L.
   [DNLM: 1. Spina Bifida—therapy.   WE 730 C737]
RJ496.S74C66 1991 617.3'75—dc20
DNLM/DLC
for Library of Congress   90-15108 CIP

Direct all inquires to CRC Press, Inc., 2000 Corporate Blvd., N.W., Boca Raton, Florida,
33431.

© 1991 by CRC Press, Inc.

International Standard Book Number 0-8493-0151-3

Library of Congress Card Number 90-15108
Printed in the United States

INTRODUCTION

As medicine moves from total ignorance of the management of spina bifida due to its near universal mortality to an era where this common condition has become a major public health problem, understanding the complex nature of this malformation is constantly and rapidly evolving. The purpose of the present work is to provide a comprehensive and current review of the management of the infant and child with spina bifida that is useful for a variety of readers, including physicians in various specialties, nurses, therapists, personnel providing care in multidisciplinary clinics, family members, and individuals with this condition.

What is Spina Bifida?

Spina bifida literally means "spine in two parts" or "open spine". Within this definition are contained many birth defects, including spina bifida occulta. This "hidden" form of spina bifida simply refers to an incomplete closure of the spinous process in a lower lumbar or sacral vertebral segment and may be found as an incidental radiographic finding in 15% of the population. Most cases of spina bifida occulta are innocuous and unassociated with neurologic deficits, orthopedic abnormalities, or genetic implications.

Some forms of spina bifida occulta, especially when associated with cutaneous stigmata such as midline dimples, hemangiomata, hairy patches, or subcutaneous lipomas, may indicate a variety of abnormal spinal cord formations. Those so-called occult dysraphic states such as diastematomyelia, intraspinal dermoid, and lipomyelomeningocele may be associated with neurological deficits and may require surgical intervention to correct the abnormality or to detether the spinal cord.

For the purpose of this work, however, spina bifida refers to spina bifida cystica, alternately called spina bifida aperta. Cystica refers to the apparent cyst on the back of the newborn with this condition. Aperta (open) refers to the obvious nature of the lesion in the newborn period. Spina bifida is one of the open neural-tube defects that include anencephaly and various types of encephaloceles. Depending on the genetic makeup of the population, spina bifida occurs between one and three times for each 1000 live births. The cause of spina bifida is thought to be multifactorial with both genetic and environmental factors interacting to cause the malformation. Recent information has stressed the importance of maternal nutrition in the production of spina bifida. Early use of prenatal vitamins containing folic acid leads to a dramatic decline in the incidence of spina bifida.

In a more holistic sense, however, spina bifida as a term derived from the abnormality of the bony spine defines an extensive, interacting complex of abnormalities that are, to a greater or lesser degree, shared by all affected patients and dealt with by these individuals, their families, and their medical caretakers. All or almost all will harbor the Arnold-Chiari malformation (described in

Chapter 4), which is only occasionally symptomatic. Between 70 and 90% have hydrocephalus. All will have bowel and bladder abnormalities, although with new techniques, bowel and bladder continence is becoming a realistic goal for most individuals with spina bifida. The majority of affected individuals will have orthopedic difficulties ranging from clubfoot deformities to spinal deformities. All of these problems are described in detail later in this volume.

Synonyms

As seen throughout this book, spina bifida has many synonyms that are used more or less interchangeably. Myelomeningocele and meningomyelocele are the most frequently used. Rather than emphasizing the bony opening in the spine as spina bifida does, these terms emphasize the actual abnormality of the spinal cord. *Meningo* refers to the meningeal coverings over the spinal cord and brain. *Cele* refers to the cyst. As pointed out several times in this work, the cyst is an envelope. Its inferior portion is the dura mater, and its superior aspect is a combination of arachnoid and neural placode. Finally, *myelo* refers to the spinal cord. Meningomyelocele, a term used frequently throughout this work, implies a cyst involving the spinal cord and meninges. These terms are used interchangeably throughout the text.

Myelodysplasia refers to the maldevelopment of the spinal cord and is often used to describe the condition. Dysraphism is a generic term for abnormalities of the formation of the central nervous system. The word derives from the median raphe, which is the dorsal indentation in the spinal cord where the neural tube has fused.

What is Not Here

This book emphasizes the treatment of the infant, child, and adolescent with spina bifida. Valve-regulated shunts, first placed in the early 1950s, were not available for general use before 1960. At that time, the population of children with spina bifida began to age, but the mortality from renal failure and shunt malfunction was still quite high. Only now are significant numbers of adults with spina bifida being treated. As adults, these patients are no longer covered by services provided to crippled children, and their care is often sporadic and rarely provided in multidisciplinary clinics. The rules for management and surgical indications may be similar for both the growing child and the adult, but only the systematic evaluation of a large group of adults treated with this malformation will allow firm recommendations to be made. Too little information is available to write about the comprehensive management of the adult with spina bifida. This topic remains one of the biggest challenges in the management of the growing spina bifida population.

THE EDITOR

Harold L. Rekate, M.D., is Chief of Pediatric Neurology at the Barrow Neurological Institute in Phoenix, Arizona, and Clinical Professor of Neurosurgery at the University of Arizona in Tucson.

Dr. Rekate graduated from Duke University in Durham, NC, in 1966 with a degree in chemistry. He obtained his medical degree from the Medical College of Virginia in Richmond in 1970. He trained in general surgery and then in neurosurgery at the University Hospitals of Cleveland, OH, at Case Western Reserve University. Upon completion of his training, he joined the faculty at Case Western Reserve University School of Medicine in both the Departments of Surgery (Neurosurgery) and Pediatrics.

Dr. Rekate is a Fellow of the American College of Surgeons and the American College of Pediatrics. He is a member of the American Association of Neurological Surgeons, Congress of Neurological Surgeons, International Society of Pediatric Neurosurgery, American Society of Pediatric Neurosurgeons, and the Neurological Society of America.

He has a long history of working with children with spina bifida and their families. He served as the Director of Child's Brain Center at Rainbow Babies and Children's Hospital in Cleveland and as neurosurgeon to its Birth Defect Center from 1978 until he moved to Phoenix in 1985. Dr. Rekate has been recognized for his treatment and education of spina bifida by the Spina Bifida Association of Southern Arizona and the Arizona Spina Bifida Association and has addressed the National Convention of the Spina Bifida Association of America on two occasions. Dr. Rekate was selected to be a member of the faculty of the Annual European Pediatric Neurosurgical Course.

Dr. Rekate's research activities concern the pathophysiology and treatment of hydrocephalus. This research has led to grants from the National Institutes of Health and the National Aeronautics and Space Administration. He has published over 50 articles on pediatric neurosurgical subjects.

ACKNOWLEDGMENTS

Many people deserve thanks for making this book possible. First and foremost, thanks go to individuals who have spina bifida and to their families. All that we know of the medical conditions described within this volume we have learned from you. More importantly, much of what we know of the human spirit, of courage, and of strength, we have learned from you. The Spina Bifida Association of America, especially the chapters in Cleveland, Phoenix, and Tucson, was originally perceived as threatening by the medical caretakers of children with spina bifida because they continually asked questions and sought other opinions. It did not take long, however, to realize how an informed consumer of medical care could be our greatest ally in the care of patients with this complex malformation.

Special thanks go to Dr. Frank E. Nulsen, one of the developers of the valve-regulated shunt who established one of the country's first comprehensive spina bifida management clinics at Rainbow Babies' and Children's Hospital in Cleveland. Patient loyalty to this innovative physician resulted in the formation of a large volume clinic with a stable population of children and young adults with spina bifida whose progress was thoroughly documented. The ongoing study of this patient population became a living laboratory from which many of the conclusions expressed here are derived.

The important role played by the late Dr. David E. Richards cannot be underestimated. Through his influence, emphasis changed from *spina bifida patients* to *Patrick* and *Clara* and *Scott*. He taught surgical techniques and also how to talk to patients — but most importantly — how to listen.

The Editorial Office of the Barrow Neurological Institute, directed by Shelley A. Kick, Ph.D., and assisted by Ms. Sarah De Alva and Ms. Karen Sellers, was essential in the preparation of this work. Their patience and support are deeply appreciated. The help of Mr. Steven Harrison, BNI Medical Illustrator, and Ms. Pamela Smith, BNI Medical Photographer, is also gratefully acknowledged. And, of course, the book could not have been produced without the commitment of CRC Press and its devoted personnel.

Last, but surely not least, I thank my wife, to whom the book is dedicated. She has encouraged me — heedless of the stress — not only throughout this project, but throughout my career and life.

To Mary Lou, who encourages me in all things

CONTRIBUTORS

Robert B. Bailey, M.D.
Suite 401
3411 North Fifth Avenue
Phoenix, Arizona

Lynda Dallyn, M.S.W.
Children's Rehabilitation Service
St. Joseph's Hospital and Medical
  Center
Phoenix, Arizona

Morris S. Dixon, Jr., M.D.
Department of Pediatrics
Lakewood Hospital
Lakewood, Ohio

Carolynne Garrison-Jones, Ph.D.
Children's Rehabilitation Service
St. Joseph's Hospital
  and Medical Center
Phoenix, Arizona

May L. Griebel, M.D.
Division of Pediatric Neurology
Arkansas Children's Hospital
Little Rock, Arkansas

Jack K. Mayfield, M.D.
Pediatric Orthopaedics and Spine
Surgery, Ltd.
Phoenix, Arizona

W. Jerry Oakes, M.D.
Department of Surgery and
  Pediatrics
Duke University Medical Center
Durham, North Carolina

R. Craig Pomatto, C.P.O.
SW Orthotic & Prosthetic
  Rehabilitation
Phoenix, Arizona

Harold L. Rekate, M.D.
Chief, Pediatric Neurosurgery
Barrow Neurological Insitute
Phoenix, Arizona

Theodore J. Tarby, M.D., Ph.D.
Department of Child Neurology
Barrow Neurological Institute
Phoenix, Arizona

Gordon Worley, M.D.
Department of Pediatrics
Duke University Medical Center
Durham, North Carolina

TABLE OF CONTENTS

Chapter 1

NEUROSURGICAL MANAGEMENT OF THE NEWBORN WITH SPINA BIFIDA

Harold L. Rekate

TABLE OF CONTENTS

I. ASSESSMENT

Initial neurological assessment of the newborn with spina bifida is extremely important because it is the best estimate of the child's potential motor, and to a somewhat lesser extent, higher cognitive performance. The assessment defines the biological substrate of the child's nervous system deranged by myelomeningocele and the Chiari II malformation. The recurrent theme of this chapter is that the examiner should, after this examination, be able to offer a reasonable prediction of the child's motor potential throughout life.

Implicit in this chapter is the corollary that if the child is not achieving the biological potential defined by the initial assessment, something is occurring that is probably correctable. This factor must be actively pursued diagnostically and treated aggressively. Spina bifida is a static abnormality of the developing nervous system, but produces a nervous system (both brain and spinal cord) that is extremely sensitive to injury from a variety of causes which are described below.

A. Physiologic and Neurologic Examination

After the child has been stabilized and transferred to the neonatal intensive care unit, a general physical and neurological assessment should be performed. Optimally, the child should be assessed by a neurosurgeon and a pediatrician, both of whom will continue to be involved in the child's care throughout the hospital stay. This joint assessment is more thorough and is especially important in assuring the family that they are receiving the same information from each caretaker and that the information is as accurate as possible. Because of the perceived urgency of the situation, the examinations should be performed simultaneously, if possible. Thorough and frequent communication among the pediatrician, neurosurgeons, and nursing staff is essential in minimizing confusion in the minds of the family at this stressful time.

1. Head and Neck

The examination of the head and neck in newborns carries unique considerations. Hydrocephalus, defined by the need for shunting in 70 to 90% of children born with spina bifida and defined by ventriculomegaly on imaging studies in at least 90% of children born with spina bifida, is rarely overt at birth. Unless the hydrocephalus is complicated by a secondary aqueductal stenosis, the cerebrospinal fluid (CSF) communicates with the lumbar theca and decompresses into the myelomeningocele sac. Because of the lack of the pressure head of CSF to act with the growing brain to expand the skull, the children may be born with a mild relative microcephaly or may be born with a normal head circumference despite moderate ventriculomegaly.

The shape of the skull in newborns with spina bifida (and therefore the Chiari II malformation) will be unusual. The posterior fossa is extremely small, and this reverses the normally rounded configuration of the occipital bone. If

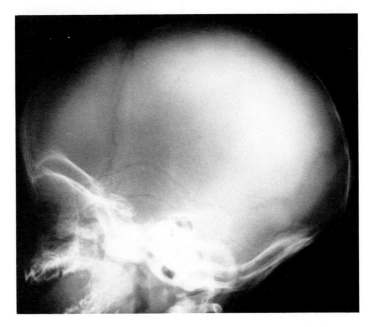

A

FIGURE 1. Comparison of plain radiographs of the skull of a normal newborn (A) with that of a child with spina bifida (B). The film in B demonstrates a mild degree of Lückenschädl and reversal of the normal curve of the basiocciput.

hydrocephalus is present, even if not overt, this curve-reversal can lead to a prominent parieto-occipital bossing. Secondarily, this may cause a more posteriorly tipped forehead.

The lacunar skull deformity, visible on the radiographs of nearly all children born with spina bifida, may lead to abnormalities of skull shape, particularly scalloping and flaring of the posterior and superior portions of the frontal bone, giving some of these children an initial mildly trigonencephalic appearance. The lacunar skull deformity, which has been referred to as *lückenschädl*, is the presence of noncalcified areas of cyst within the membranous bone portions of the calvarium. When prominent, this may be associated with palable areas of softening of the skull itself. With growth of the skull and regardless of whether the child has been shunted, these cystic areas will disappear — usually within the first 6 months (Figure 1).[1]

Many children with spina bifida begin life with a tendency to maintain their heads in a markedly retroflexed position, presumably reflecting the traction on the upper cervical nerve roots created by the Arnold-Chiari malformaation (described in Chapter 4). In most children, this condition resolves or becomes intermittent after the first 4 months. In others, however, it may be the first sign of progressive difficulties in brain stem function associated with the Chiari crisis or symptomatic Arnold-Chiari malformation.

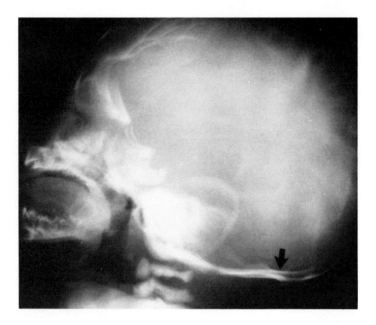

FIGURE 1B.

2. Chest and Abdomen

Several concerns relative to the examination of the chest and abdomen of the child with spina bifida are noteworthy. Presumably because the anlage of the ribs is being formed at the same time that the central nervous system (CNS) is being affected by the development of myelomeningocele, rib abnormalities are quite common in these children. Usually these abnormalities simply result in radiographically visible rib fusions and increased spaces between ribs (Figure 2). In severe cases, however, partial flail chest or restrictions of chest movements can be seen clinically. When severe spinal deformity is present, the shape of the chest cage may be a bizarre reflection of the deformity of the entire structure of the thorax.

In children with lesions at the thoracolumbar level, the abdomen may appear very protuberant. This appearance results from the lack of development of the abdominal musculature. Intra-abdominal difficulties often found in these children, such as renal anomalies or hydronephrosis, are rarely discernible on physical examination.

3. Examination of the Back

The most dramatic portion of the physical examination of the newborn with myelomeningocele (spina bifida cystica) is the overt lesion of the back. The lesion of myelomeningocele always contains certain elements that can be viewed during the initial examination. The central feature is the neural placode, the remnant of the spinal cord presenting through the spinal and soft tissue

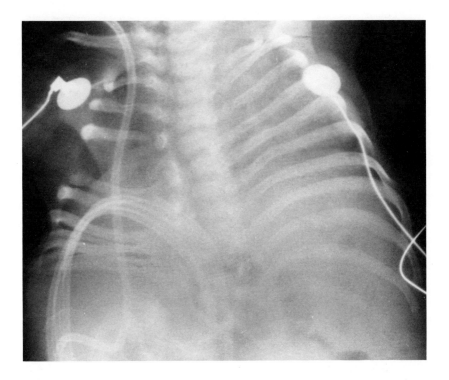

FIGURE 2. Plain radiograph of a child with a thoracolumbar myelomeningocele demonstrating severe rib abnormalities.

hernia. It is contiguous rostrally with the spinal cord within the spine. It is normally rust-red and can be quite small and difficult to see if very broad over many segments (Figure 3).

Surrounding the neural placode and fused both to it and to the surrounding skin is a translucent or transparent membrane representing the arachnoid. The skin surrounding and fused with the arachnoid may be humped up in and around the sac containing CSF, or it may be tightly adherent to the underlying soft issues. If the sac is ruptured (i.e., empty of CSF), the placode will be lying in the open bifid remnants of the spinal canal. If no rupture has occurred, the cyst may rise 3 or 4 cm from the surface of the child's back with the neural placode at the apex.

In some cases, the neural placode is not visible and the neurologic examination is normal. These findings led to the diagnosis of meningocele. This condition must be exceedingly rare. These children should be followed carefully and have magnetic resonance imaging (MRI) studies looking for the Chiari II malformation and for signs of spinal cord tethering.

Careful attention should be paid to the dimensions of the lesion and its anatomic location with respect to the sacrum, iliac crests, and lower rib cage. Specific anatomic levels relative to myotomes cannot be discerned on the basis

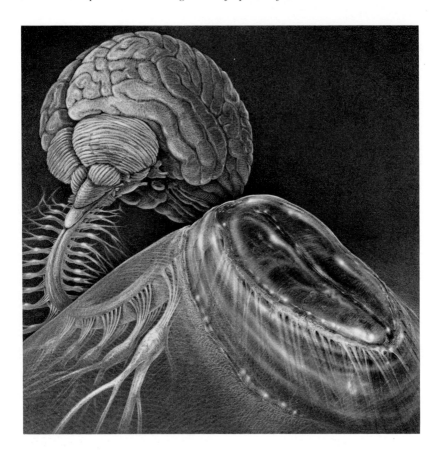

FIGURE 3. Artist's concept of the relationship of the newborn myelomeningocele to the spine and nerve roots. (From the cover photograph: *BNI Q.*, 4(4), 1988. With permission.)

of the examination of the back, but functional levels that are important predictors of the child's functional ability can usually be inferred from the location of the lesion. In general, a lesion limited entirely to the sacrum in the area of the intergluteal fold can be referred to as a sacral level lesion. A lesion in this location will generally spare all or most of the musculature involved in locomotion and will only be associated with difficulties with bowel and bladder control. A lesion centered at or about the level of the iliac crest will be referred to as a lumbosacral level lesion. Besides bowel and bladder dysfunction, these patients will have some paralysis of the musculature of the ankles and may have mildly unbalanced hips. These children can be expected to be community ambulators requiring short leg (AFO) braces and/or surgical stabilization of the ankles. When the lesion is above the iliac crest but below the ribs, it is referred to as a lumbar level lesion, implying complete paralysis of the ankles but retained knee extension and marked weakness in knee flexion and hip extension. These children will likely require extensive surgery to stabilize the hip, but most can be expected to remain ambulators with braces and crutches. Above this level, the lesions are referred to as thoracolumbar or thoracic. They may have some hip flexor function in the lower extremities. In preteen years, using extensive bracing and crutches, these children can stand and get around. However, by the time they are teenagers, the energy requirements for ambulating their larger bodies nearly always leads to the use of wheelchairs for mobility.

The physical examination of the back itself will reveal the extent of the opening of the spine and may show significant spinal deformities. A rather common, though extremely severe form of spinal deformity in children with thoracolumbar or high lumbar level lesions is myelokyphosis or gibbus. This anomaly is an unstable reversal of the normal lumbar curve that lacks any bony or soft tissue elements posteriorly. The presence of this anomaly makes repairing the myelomeningocele more difficult than usual. If repaired using normal techniques, the child is left with marked difficulty in maintaining an erect posture for sitting or standing in orthoses. These problems are discussed in greater detail with the repair of lesions and under the section on orthopedic management.

4. The Lower Extremities

The examination of the lower extremities, except in the case of children with pure sacral level lesions, will frequently reveal deformities, particularly of the ankles but also often of the foreleg and knees. These deformities often mirror the degree of neurologic deficit *in utero*. For example, a foot deformed in a slightly dorsiflexed and internally rotated position can be presumed to have had a functioning anterior tibial muscle (L4) *in utero* that was unopposed either by peroneii (L5) or gastrocnemius (S1). Frequently, however, the lesion level predicted by the foot deformity underestimates the degree of involvement. For instance, in the above example at the time of birth, the L4 muscles may not be working either.

The bony structures of the infants are extremely plastic at this time. Especially at the lumbosacral level, it is vital to correct the arthrogryposis early to allow the children to wear shoes and to stand correctly. Serial casting, therefore, should normally begin in the neonatal intensive care unit or immediately after discharge.

5. The Neurologic Examination

The newborn's neurologic examination is difficult because of the infant's passive nature. The examination is unavoidably subjective to a degree, and different examiners will frequently map different sensory examinations. It is also difficult to maintain infants with a large, full myelomeningocele on their back to examine the sensation of the anterior legs and abdomen.

The examination of the head was described earlier. The cranial nerve examination is extremely important in these children because it is highly likely that they will have a cranial nerve abnormality during development. Eye movements are of particular interest. These children often have unilateral or bilateral palsies of the abducens of various degrees, even without overt hydrocephalus. Other abnormalities of occular motility can be seen. Trigeminal and facial nerve function, as well as statoacoustic nerve function, are rarely involved. The lower cranial nerves (discussed later), IX through XII, are not intracranial structures in the Chiari II malformation but actually exit the brain stem within the cervical canal. Drooling and an absent gag reflex signal difficulties with the glossopharyngeal (IX) and vagal (X) nerves. Abnormal vagal nerve function can present as stridor with bilateral paralysis of the vocal cords that requires intubation. Often tracheostomy is needed when this condition cannot be reversed. Retropulsion of the neck and weakness of the shoulder shrug indicate difficulty with the spinal accessory cranial nerve (XI). The tongue (hypoglossal, XII) should be examined for atrophy or fasciculations.

The motor examination is performed by stimulating and observing the child's patterns of movement. While the upper extremities may weaken from compression of the brain stem or syringomyelia later in childhood, motor function is usually normal in the newborn. Examining the lower extremities of children born with myelomeningocele will reveal the actual motor level of retained ability indicative of the child's level of potential functioning. For example, retained ability to plantar flex the feet indicates retention of the S1 myotome; foot eversion indicates retention of L5; foot inversion indicates retention of L4; knee extension indicates retention of L2 or L3; and hip flexion indicates retention of L1. This system emphasizes the concept of *ability* as opposed to *disability*.[2] Significant differences between the right and left legs are common; in such cases, both are referred to, e.g., L4 on the right and S1 on the left.

The sensory examination of the lower extremities is even more subject to asymmetry in children with myelomeningocele than is the motor system. Also, a thorough sensory examination is extremely difficult in these children because of their paucity of responses to stimulation. The pin-prick examination is begun in areas most likely to be anesthetic (e.g., perineal area) and extended proximally until the child appears to be made uncomfortable by the pin; then, the dermatome is recorded. At this point, the child is comforted until quiet, and the same procedure is performed on the other side.

The reflex examination is performed in a routine fashion on the newborn and the deep tendon reflexes of the involved muscles are characteristically absent. Spasticity, so important in the later assessment of children with myelomeningocele is almost never present in newborns. The remainder of the neurologic examination is unreliable at this time because the child cannot cooperate in the assessment.

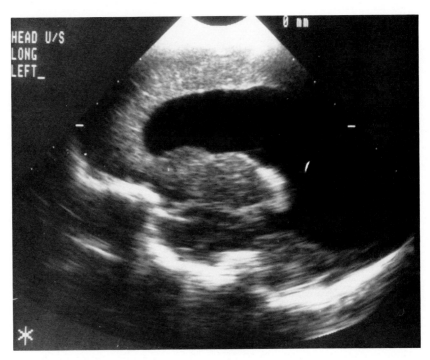

FIGURE 4. Ultrasound study showing ventriculomegaly in a newborn with a lumbosacral myelomeningocele.

B. Radiologic Assessment

No radiologic assessment is absolutely required before repair of the myelomeningocele; however, if convenient, some studies seem indicated. Ventricular size should be assessed. This is most easily obtained in newborns by using real-time ultrasonography. The procedure can be obtained in the neonatal intensive care unit and provides an adequate view of the size and shape of the lateral ventricle (Figure 4). Actual anatomy of the Chiari malformation is best defined using MRI, but the elegance of such a study is rarely required before closure of the back lesion, making the transport of the child and performance of the study easier.

Plain skull radiographs will reveal lückenschädl, a reversal of the curve of the occipital bone: small posterior fossa and sellar abnormalities characteristic of the Chiari II malformation.[1] None of the information will have an appreciable impact on management decisions in the first few days of the child's life.

Plain radiographs of the spine will show the extent of the open spinal defect and may reveal a significant spinal deformity. The presence of a myelokyphosis or gibbus may not be obvious on physical examination; when present, it may signify that the lesion will be more difficult to close and may even require the assistance of a plastic surgeon or a decision to resect the kyphus at the time of repair.

II. NEUROSURGICAL PRINCIPLES

Whether to treat children born with severe myelomeningocele is often intensely and passionately debated. What is meant by nontreatment is also a concept that changes. The arguments deserve some comment. Before valve-regulated shunts were developed in the early 1950s,[3] this problem was moot because most of these children died from progressive hydrocephalus, with or without repair of the lesion. During the early era of shunting, many children were treated with back closure and early shunting. Lorber reported that a series of untreated children with myelomeningocele showed a correlation of poor intellect with hydrocephalus overt at birth, high-level paraplegia, presence of myelokyphosis, and neonatal asphyxia, or other severe congenital abnormalities. He suggested that children showing any two of these markers of poor outcome should be selected for nontreatment.[4] Afterward, he reported an impressive improvement in outcomes in a series of children in whom these criteria were applied.[5]

In Lorber's own nonselected series, 20% of the children who would have been selected for nontreatment had IQs in the normal or near-normal range. This was true in every reported series of children with myelomeningocele and led other investigators to attempt to refine the criteria to save those children who were not doomed to severely subnormal intelligence. A variety of criteria were added, such as the presence of lückenschädl on plain skull radiographs or other radiologic abnormalities.[6] These studies failed to refine further Lorber's criteria and presumed that something intrinsic in the diffuse cortical abnormalities of the Chiari II malformation (e.g., polymicrogyria, cortical ectasias, hydrocephalus) precluded normal intelligence. Not until the work of McLone et al.[7,8] was it realized that mental subnormality in the context of the Chiari II malformation is preventable by treating hydrocephalus and ventriculitis.[7,8] This work has subsequently been supported by others.[9]

The fate of children selected for nontreatment becomes extremely important because prolonged delays in treatment of the back lesion may lead to ventriculitis and subsequent intellectual deterioration. In one study, as many as 50% of the children selected for nontreatment (i.e., no closure of the back lesion and no antibiotics) did not die either because the back lesion granulated over and the ventriculomegaly stabilized.[54] Unstated, but implicit from the work of McLone and others, is that a significant number of these children will be left more severely impaired than chidren who are aggressively treated.[7-9] In contrast, another study has shown that 90% of children selected for nontreatment die within 1 year.[10]

The ethics of allowing damaged newborns to die is considered elsewhere.[11,12] Children with myelomeningocele may not die when they receive less aggressive treatment, but they may suffer severe CNS injury from the non-treatment. For the purposes of this discussion, this fact compels recommending early aggressive treatment of all newborns with myelomeningocele.

A. Management of the Lesion of the Back

Having decided that essentially all children born with myelomeningocele should have the lesion repaired, the next discussion concerns the initial management of the lesion and the timing of the intervention. Early reports of improved neurologic condition after rushing the child to surgery have not been confirmed.[13-16] In fact, some studies show as good results with delayed surgery.[17] One study reports improved overall outcome with rather prolonged delays in attention to back closure.[18-20] Hard data on how to treat these back lesions before closure are difficult to find. Therefore, it seems reasonable to place a sterile dressing on the lesion and to place the child on meningitic doses of antibiotics such as ampicillin and gentamycin while awaiting closure. While surgery as a compelling emergency may not be necessary, the possibility of the open neural tube defect becoming colonized with bacteria suggests that the back should be repaired as soon as practical and within 48 to 72 h.

1. The Anatomy of Myelomeningocele

The surface anatomy of the myelomeningocele lesion was described in the section on physical examination and in Figure 3. Figure 5 shows the lesion in cross section. Understanding the anatomical relationships is crucial to closing the defect properly. At the apex of the cystic structure is the flat neural placode. At the edge of the placode, the remnants of the arachnoid insert in the area of the entry zone of the nerve root. From this junction, the nerve roots, which are mostly nonfunctional, descend to exit through neural foramina located ventrally. The arachnoid membrane then traverses laterally to fuse with the skin at the lateral reaches of the lesion. Forming a third leg of this tripod directed medially and ventrally is the distended dura mater, which is loosely adherent to the underlying soft tissue of the back and densely adherent to the bony structures of the bifid spine. Rostrally, the dura forms a tube and the neural placode also begins to form an internal tube that leads to the functional spinal cord within the closed spine.[21]

2. Standard Techniques for Closure of Myelomeningocele

The primary purpose of closing a myelomeningocele is to seal the CNS from bacteria entering via CSF. Another goal of closure is to prevent the secondary tethering that occurs in these children. Finally, it is essential that no skin element become buried in the repair because of the possibility of developing an expanding dermoid.

The first step in the repair of the myelomeningocele is isolating the neural placode while salvaging the nerve roots. After prepping the child from the high thoracic area to the gluteal fold and from table to table, the child is draped

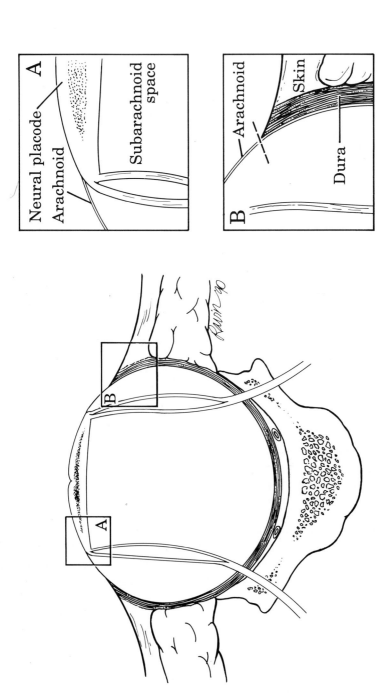

FIGURE 5. Cross-section of myelomeningocele sac demonstrating two tripods where distinct tissues come together. One tripod involves the skin, arachnoid, and dura; the other involves the arachnoid, neural placode, and nerve roots. (From McLaurin, R. L., *Contemp. Neurosurg.*, 6, 1, 1984. With permission.)

appropriately. This extensive prepping is needed in case rotational or bipedicle flaps are necessary for skin closure. The skin incision is circumferential around the lesion to maintain as much viable skin as possible. Meticulous hemostasis is essential and most small myelomeningoceles can be repaired without transfusion.

Hemostats are used to hold up the dissected skin and arachnoid, and the skin hooks are saved for countertraction on the skin. After this circumferential incision is made, the arachnoid is lifted and the nerve roots are teased medially from the arachnoid to the site of exit from the neural placode. At this point, the remnants of skin and arachnoid are sharply removed from the neural placode.

While little experimental evidence supports its use, the next step recommended by McLone[22] is creating a neural tube from the placode by inverting it and suturing it with nonabsorbable sutures. There is hope that beside being a biologically correct step, recreating the neural tube will prevent later tethering.

Next, the dura is dissected from the underlying soft tissue. The dissection begins at the confluence of the tripod of arachnoid, skin, and dura (Figure 6) and proceeds medially and bilaterally and is simple until the bony ridges of the bifid spine are encountered. Here, dissection becomes extremely difficult, and the repair can be jeopardized by holes formed from attempting to dissect the dura from the underlying bone. If the spine is widely bifid and the dura is insufficient to permit a watertight closure, the surgeon has two options. It is often possible to remove the top edge of the cartilaginous portion of the spine with the dura by using a No. 15 blade, thereby preventing a rent and allowing more dissection. If the dura is still insufficient to close, the use of graft material from either the child's own lumbodorsal fascia or by way of a lyophilized dural graft may be used. In contrast, if the dural dissection has left the surgeon with redundant dura, an overlapping flap may be created giving an approximation of a two-layered closure.

The dural closure must be watertight and should be checked by having the anesthetist perform a Valsalva maneuver to insure patency. If possible, the dural closure should also allow the newly created neural tube to be surrounded by CSF in the hope of preventing later tethering.[22] The next step is to attempt to gain a second layer of closure using lumbodorsal fascia. The overlying skin is dissected from the underlying musculature. In the lumbar region, the lumbodorsal fascia is well developed across most of the back. It can be sharply dissected from the underlying musculature and closed in the midline. In low lumbar and sacral lesions, the lumbodorsal fascia thins and disappears in the area of the gluteal musculature; this layer cannot be closed in this location without grafting.

The final step in the closure of small and moderate lesions is the skin closure. Using blunt dissection, the skin is dissected from the underlying fascia and musculature; skin hooks are used in an attempt to approximate the skin edges. Usually, the skin is approximated bringing it from a lateral to medial

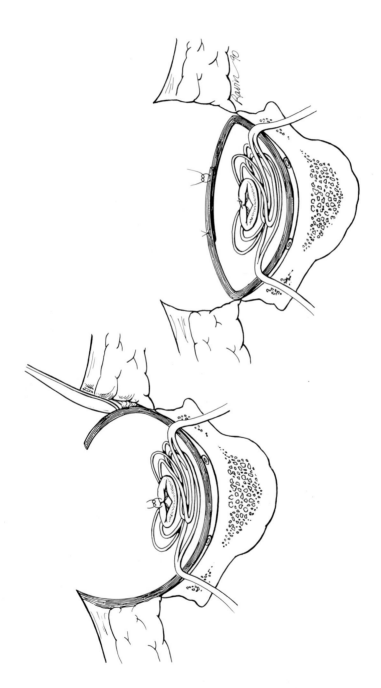

FIGURE 6.   Drawing of dissection of the dura from the underlying soft tissue to obtain a watertight closure.

direction; occasionally, it is best approximated rostrocaudally. The skin is often closed under mild tension, but if the edges are blanched at the time approximation, it is unlikely that they will remain viable. Then, some form of flap should be used to prevent necrosis of the skin edges over the dural repair.

After repair of the myelomeningocele, the child should be maintained in a prone or lateral decubitus position to prevent pressure on the repair. If a shunt or external ventricular drainage has not been performed, the child should be maintained in a head-down position to prevent the hydrostatic pressure of the CSF from jeopardizing the repair.

3. Closure of Large Myelomeningocele Defects

Frequently, it is not possible to close the skin primarily without undue tension. In these situations, skin flaps or myocutaneous flaps are necessary. For most defects the use of bilateral bipedicle flaps (lateral relaxing incisions) are adequate to achieve a good closure.

To perform this, the skin is bluntly dissected from the underlying soft tissues. Longitudinal incisions parallel to the spine are made on either side at the posterior axillary line, creating long skin bridges on either side of the defect with blood supply derived from both ends of the flap. These bilateral bipedicle flaps are then approximated in the midline. This technique allows excellent, tensionless closure over large defects.[23-25]

What to do with the lateral area of skin back is a matter of some controversy. Immediate closure tends to add tension to the medial suture line and is rarely indicated. Immediate skin grafting from the buttocks has also been advocated. It usually is sufficient to allow the areas to epithelialize on their own using wet to dry dressing changes two times per day for debridement.

Especially in the context of the thoracolumbar kyphotic deformity or gibbus, bringing skin edges over sharp bony prominences may result in skin necrosis with secondary exposure of the previously closed neural placode. In these situations, it is often advisable to seek the assistance of experienced plastic surgeons for the performance of myocutaneous flaps to increase the cushion over the bony prominences. These flaps require a thorough understanding of the blood supply of the latissimus dorsi muscles and occasionally large volumes of blood loss can be expected.[26-28]

The presence of a kyphus or gibbus not only makes myelomeningocele closure extremely difficult, it interferes with the positioning and bracing of the young child. For these reasons Sharrard[29] and Reigel[30,31] have advocated resection of the kyphus with primary spinal fusion at the time of myelomeningocele closure. They do well in the immediate postoperative period, but between the ages of 2 and 10, a progressive recurrent kyphosis can be identified.[30] The author has performed initial kyphectomy on two newborns in association with orthopedics. The procedure is not difficult and is well tolerated by the babies. The children have been managed in a "clam shell" orthosis postoperatively. These children have not been followed long enough for the late development of kyphosis but are much better suited for their needed bracing and sitting than are children with a retained kyphus. The place of early kyphectomy in these children is still undefined.

III. MANAGEMENT OF HYDROCEPHALUS IN THE NEWBORN

Most children born with myelomeningocele will have associated hydrocephalus. The actual percentage of children partially depends on the *working* definition. If hydrocephalus is defined as any degree of ventriculomegaly, then <5% of these infants are spared hydrocephalus. While some children born with myelomeningocele have overt hydrocephalus (presumably from secondary aqueductal stenosis) most are born with normal or slightly smaller than normal heads and normal or slightly generous ventricles. After the defect has been closed, its action as a buffer for intracranial pressure by venting CSF is lost, and ventriculomegaly and craniomegaly begin and progress.

In most infants, the need for shunting is quickly apparent; however, in 20 to 30%, the degree of ventriculomegaly is only mild to moderate and the rate of head growth tends to jump initially and to follow normal patterns. Significant controversy exists about how to select patients with ventriculomegaly who would benefit from a shunt. Before a surgical decision can be made, the special nature of hydrocephalus in this condition must first be understood.

A. The Etiology of Hydrocephalus in Myelomeningocele

All or nearly all children born with myelomeningocele harbor the Arnold-Chiari II malformation. In general, the anatomy of this condition is discussed elsewhere in this volume (Chapters 2 and 4). However, it is important to the pathophysiology of hydrocephalus in this condition and must be discussed here briefly. Figure 7 is a schematic representation of the CSF pathways in normal individuals. CSF is produced within the ventricular system. It arises from two sources: from an energy-dependent production by the choroid plexuses and as a passive bulk flow of CSF from brain extracellular fluid into the ventricular system.[32] CSF then passes through a series of intracranial gates (foramen of Monro, aqueduct of Sylvius, foramina of Luschka and Magendie) to exit into the cisterna magna, where it freely communicates with the spinal and cortical subarachnoid spaces. From there, it is absorbed into the venous system through specialized organs, the arachnoid granulations.[33]

Pathologic obstruction to the flow along this pathway causes hydrocephalus and backs up the flow of CSF proximal to the obstruction. This increases the size of the ventricles and usually intracranial pressure. If, however, the skull is still easily distensible as in the newborn or if the brain is abnormally compliant as in the newborn with an incompletely myelinated nervous system or in the

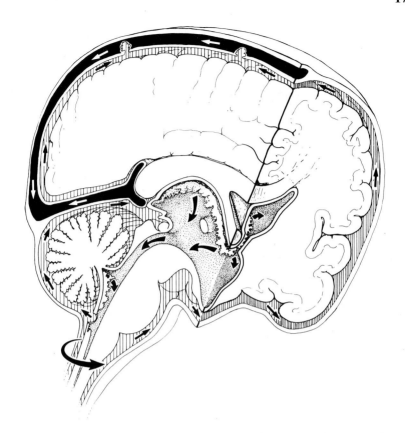

FIGURE 7. Cerebrospinal fluid pathways in a normal patient. (From Rekate, H. and Olivero, W., in *Hydrocephalus: Concepts in Neurosurgery*, Vol. 3, Scott, R. M., Ed., Williams & Wilkins, Baltimore, 1990, 11. With permission.)

aged brain, then ventricles can dilate with little, if any, increase in intracranial pressure.[34,35]

Four interactions appear to cause hydrocephalus in association with the Chiari II malformation, specifically caused by distortion in the anatomy.

1. Position of the Outlet Foramina of the Fourth Ventricle

As Figure 8 shows, the outlet foramina of the fourth ventricle are present in the cervical canal, not in the posterior fossa. The cerebellar vermis is markedly elongated and the medulla compressed from the dorsal elongated cerebellar vermis and from the ventrocaudal position of the spinal cord. Anatomic dissections at autopsy or decompressive surgery have found dense scarring of the arachnoid at the area of the foramen of Magendie, which is also buried under the vermal peg. The foramina of Luschka are likewise present in the cervical canal, tightly encased in a dense dural band, and usually encountered at about

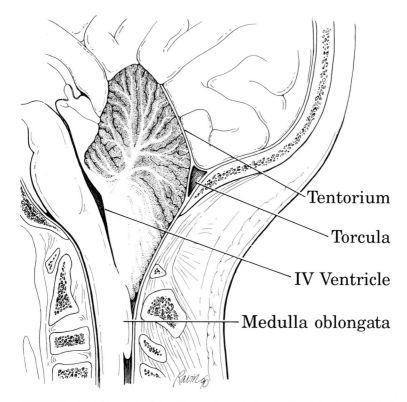

Tentorium

Torcula

IV Ventricle

Medulla oblongata

FIGURE 8. Anatomic relationships at the cervicomedullary junction in the Arnold-Chiari malformation as it relates to the etiology of hydrocephalus. (From Rekate, H. L., *BNI Q.*, 4(4), 17, 1988. With permission.)

C2. Obstruction of the outlet foramina of the fourth ventricle is the first cause of hydrocephalus associated with myelomeningocele.

2. Cork-in-the-Bottle Phenomenon

The second cause of hydrocephalus, related to the first, could be termed the cork-in-the-bottle phenomenon (Figure 9). Because the contents of the inferior portion of the posterior fossa are squeezed into the upper cervical spinal canal, this space becomes completely filled with tissue. Even if CSF could exit from the exit foramina of the fourth ventricle and reside within the spinal subarachnoid space, flow over the convexities (cortical subarachnoid space) is impeded by this cork in the spinal bottle, thereby preventing CSF from being absorbed into the venous system.

3. Secondary Aqueductal Stenosis

The entire volume of the posterior fossa is quite small in the Chiari II malformation. The tentorium is more vertical and tends to be incompetent, allowing the superior cerebellar vermis to project fairly high between the

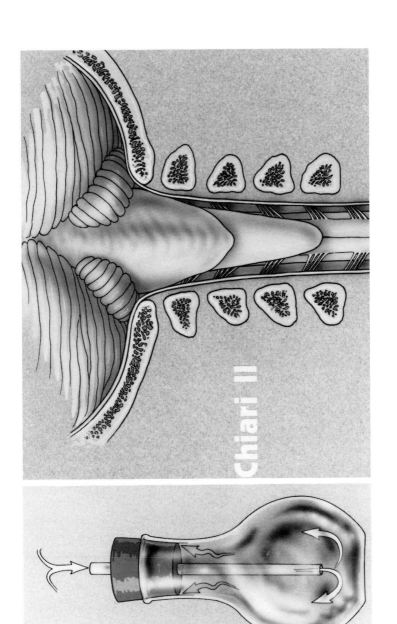

FIGURE 9. Illustration of the "cork-in-the-bottle" phenomenon as it relates to the Arnold-Chiari malformation. (From Rekate, H. L., *BNI Q*, 4(4), 17, 1988. With permission.)

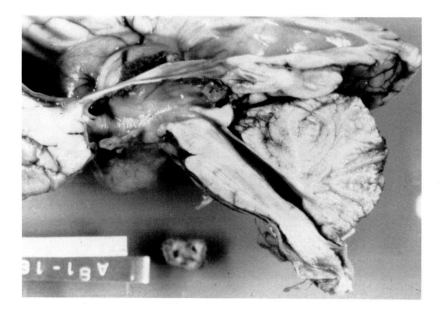

FIGURE 10.   Sagittal section of pathologic specimen showing the features of the Arnold-Chiari malformation.

occipital lobes. The entire brain stem is elongated except for the tectal beaking at the apex of the tentorium. The fourth ventricle becomes stretched or elongated with a very long course for the aqueduct. Most of the fourth ventricle lies within the cervical canal. The crowding of the structures at the apex of the posterior fossa can lead to compression of the aqueduct with proximal hydrocephalus (Figure 10). This cause of hydrocephalus can result in overt megalencephaly at birth.

4. Absorption of Cerebrospinal Fluid

Using infusions of artificial CSF, Caldarelli and colleagues have shown that children with myelomeningocele have defective CSF absorption at low infusion pressures but normal absorption at high pressures.[36] The venous structures of the posterior fossa are extremely abnormal in the context of the Chiari II malformation. The torcula and transverse sinuses frequently are present at the level of the foramen magnum. At this level, venous compression and obstruction of venous outflow would lead to the absorptive pattern described by Caldarelli, a pattern that has been shown to participate in the etiology of hydrocephalus in craniosynostosis[37] and achondroplasis[38] and may well be important in other forms of hydrocephalus.[39]

B. Management of Hydrocephalus Overt at Birth

Hydrocephalus overt at birth was one of Lorber's selection criteria for nontreatment in children with myelomeningocele.[4,5] Even in centers where aggressive treatment of myelomeningocele is the norm, the problem of managing severe, progressive, overt hydrocephalus is the subject of much discussion. The controversy occurs in two contexts: (1) when the child with hydrocephalus and myelomeningocele is diagnosed *in utero* and the hydrocephalus is rapidly advancing and (2) determining the appropriate treatment when the child presents in the delivery room with myelomeningocele and overt hydrocephalus. The ability to diagnose and even treat fetal anomalies has led to numerous discussions relative to the possibility of treating the children *in utero*. Ventriculo-amniotic shunts have been performed with mixed results. The most important question in this context is, "what is lost by waiting until the child is safe to deliver?" In this context, hard data are difficult to find, specifically as they relate to the population of children with myelomeningocele. The infantile brain is quite resilient, and in most patients, it appears that prognosis for intellectual development correlates best with the ability to reconstitute the brain after shunting rather than with the severity of the hydrocephalus at the beginning of treatment.[40] However, when hydrocephalus is overt at birth, the prognosis is often guarded. Until more experience is gained with intrauterine surgery, both from a diagnostic and technical perspective, the current recommendations for treatment depend on the gestational age and the rate of progression of the hydrocephalus. Unless hydrocephalus is massive, decisions should not be made based on a single ultrasound assessment. The rate of progression of hydrocephalus can best be assessed by an ultrasound examination at 1 to 2 week intervals.

If the hydrocephalus is not progressive, the child can be followed to term and delivered by caesarean section.[41] If, however, the hydrocephalus shows significant worsening by serial ultrasound assessments, the child should be treated as early as possible, necessitating an early delivery. Lung maturity, the limiting factor in safe early delivery and fetal viability, can be evaluated by an ultrasound-guided amniocentesis. Amniotic fluid is analyzed for lecithin to sphyngomyelin ratio. If the ratio is greater than 2, the lungs have sufficient maturity to allow normal, unassisted ventilation, and early delivery is warranted. Other tests of lung maturity include assay for phosphatidyl glycerol and desaturated phosphatidyl choline.

When a child presents with severe ventriculomegaly, megalencephaly, and an open myelomeningocele, recent authors have advocated myelomeningocele repair and ventriculoperitoneal shunting in the same procedure.[42] This practice saves the child an anesthetic and, if successful, shortens the hospital stay. Analyses of large series of patients treated in this manner have not yet been published. In my personal experience with a small series of infants treated this way, the incidence of early shunt failure and infection has been higher than in children in whom shunting has been delayed 3 to 7 d. If hydrocephalus is severe at birth, the intracranial pressure can be managed using external ventricular drainage, but this is rarely needed.

C. Surgical Decision Making: to Shunt or Not to Shunt

Most children born with myelomeningocele will need shunting. For the few for whom the decision is not straightforward, objective guidelines are needed. If there were no risks involved in the shunting procedure, then all children with ventricles larger than normal should be shunted. Studies of intellectual functioning of children with myelomeningocele have shown that children who never had a shunt, on the whole, do better intellectually than shunted children. Interpreting such retrospective studies to help make decisions on individual patients leads to difficulty because the shunted group presumably had more severe hydrocephalus initially. Whether children with ventriculomegaly and no shunt would have had better outcomes with a shunt may never be known. Performing a shunt carries risk of infection, failure, and insidious deterioration at the time of shunt failure (specifically, in children with the Chiari II malformation or myelomeningocele); therefore, the available information is assessed below to help in the decision making.

First, the biologic cost of untreated hydrocephalus must be evaluated. For children with overt hydrocephalus and increased intracranial pressure, the cost is death or rapid expansion of the head to grotesque proportions, clearly unacceptable. For these children, the decision is obvious. The natural history of untreated hydrocephalus is at least partially available and is so grim, the study can never be repeated.[43] Young and colleagues, in contrast, demonstrated that the severity of hydrocephalus before treatment was a poor predictor of intellectual attainments in shunted children. Furthermore, the post-treatment thickness of the brain at the level of the coronal suture on ventriculographic air studies was the best predictor of good intellectual outcome. Children whose post-treatment brain thickness (i.e., mantle) was more than 2.8 cm seem to fare as well as those who achieved a normal (i.e., 4.5 to 5 cm) cerebral mantle.[40] Subsequently, others used this study to define the goals of treatment for hydrocephalus children with the hope of preventing shunt dependency.[44-46]

Recent studies have tended to show that more subtle neuropsychological parameters not measured on IQ tests may be improved with normal or smaller than normal ventricles.[55] A provocative discussion by Lorber, however, relates the case of a graduate student in mathematics, who functioned normally with massive ventriculomegaly.[47] Despite the continuing controversy over the acceptable degree of hydrocephalus, the current recommendations that the mantle (i.e., the thickness of the brain at the coronal suture or foramen of Monro) be at least 3.5 cm by the age of 5 months old seem justified.[48] This 5-month cutoff was also chosen with reference to the work of Young et al., who found that when shunting was delayed beyond 5 months, the mantle was less amenable to reconstruction.[40]

The mantle, measured directly from the cranial real-time ultrasound, is the distance from the probe in the anterior fontanel to the apex of the frontal horn of the lateral ventricle in the approximate plane of the foramen of Monro. An approximation of mantle thickness can be obtained from computed tomography (CT) or magnetic resonance imaging (MRI) using the following formula:

$$M_1 = \frac{M_2 \times C_1}{\pi \times D_2}$$

where M_1 = the actual cerebral mantle, M_2 = the mantle measured from the scan, C_1 = the child's head circumference, and D_2 = the diameter of the image of the CT or MRI scan.[48] Most CT and MRI scan software permit direct measurements from the viewing/monitoring screen and make the above approximation unnecessary.

The need to establish a 3.5-cm mantle by 5 months also derives from the work of Young, who found that when treatment was delayed beyond 5 months, it was much less likely to result in the desired cerebral mantle.[40] This need should be considered only one of several criteria that must be met to allow the child to be followed without a shunt. Another criterion common to hydrocephalus children and not unique to children with myelomeningocele involves the assessment of developmental functioning. Logically, if the infant is exhibiting developmental delays, the chances for normal motor and intellectual attainment are probably diminished. Testing such as the Denver Developmental Test (DDST) is difficult to interpret in children with myelomeningocele because of the intrinsic motor difficulties associated with the defect. If the DDST is abnormal when the gross motor portion is factored out and the child has significant ventriculomegaly, then even if the 3.5 cm criterion is met, a shunt should be placed. Hard data to support the position of shunting children with mild hydrocephalus do not exist; however, the critical nature of this decision to the child's potential for a productive and independent existence leads to the conclusion that to maximize the child's potential, a shunt will guarantee that everything that can be done has been done.

Two criteria for shunting are unique to the context of the Chiari II malformation and myelomeningocele. First and most devastating is the symptomatic Chiari II malformation discussed at length elsewhere in this volume (Chapter 4). These children present with central sleep apnea and lower cranial nerve dysfunction. Because one potential etiological factor in the pathogenesis of this condition is the impact of the malformed cerebellar vermis and medulla in the cervical canal, whenever symptoms or signs relating to this syndrome are detected, a working shunt must first be placed or guaranteed. In some cases, the shunt will reverse or stabilize the condition; in others; it will progress and require later decompression. It is not, however, infrequent that performance of a shunting procedure will worsen or bring on such symptoms.

The second criterion for shunting in the myelomeningocele population is the presence of syringomyelia. Before the advent of MRI, this condition was extremely difficult to diagnose. The routine use of such studies is able to document the presence of syringomyelia before any clinical evidence of its presence. Because of the relationship of syringomyelia to hydrocephalus, the finding of syringomyelia, even in an asymptomatic patient without a shunt, implies that the child is compensating for hydrocephalus through the central canal at the expense of the spinal cord. This condition therefore requires the performance of a shunt.[49]

The above arguments seem to make a strong case for performing a shunt in all children with myelomeningocele and even mild ventriculomegaly. One caveat seems important to emphasize: shunt infection, specifically in the context of the Chiari II malformation, carries the risk of severe intellectual downgrading. The work of McLone,[7,8] which defined CNS infection rather than anatomic disorganization as the primary cause of intellectual subnormalcy in the spina bifida population, has subsequently been supported.[9] The incidence of CNS infection has been as high as 17% in newborns with spina bifida. Two thirds of these were asssociated with shunt procedures.[50] Large series of shunts report infection rates ranging from 2 to 13% per procedure.[51-53] The percentage of children with shunt infections in the context of the Chiari II malformation that will be intellectually downgraded is difficult to ascertain but would be zero if no shunt procedure were ever performed. Shunting a child with a myelomeningocele is not without risk.

D. Strategy for Hydrocephalus Surveillance

Figure 11 is the algorithm recommended for surgical decision making and follow-up of children born with myelomeningocele. As emphasized in Chapter 3, all patients born with myelomeningocele should be followed yearly throughout childhood and adolescence, preferably in the context of a multidisciplinary spina bifida clinic.

Children who have been followed over the first 5 months of life and did not require a shunt by the above criteria have not required subsequent shunting.[49] The routine use of MRI, however, may lead to a reevaluation of some children. The finding of syringomyelia on an MRI scan would require placing a shunt even with only modest hydrocephalus and no other signs of neurologic compromise. Hall et al. have shown the importance of syringomyelia as a cause of scoliosis and its reversal with shunting.[49] As discussed elsewhere, MRI has the ability to detect abnormalities of the CNS that may lead to subsequent deterioration.

Most children with hydrocephalus and spina bifida will eventually develop smaller than normal ventricular systems, and it is essential that the neurosurgeon assure that the child have at least 3.5 cm of cortical mantle. This is attainable in all but a few children with massive hydrocephalus at birth. Imaging studies (ultrasound with open fontanel, CT, or MRI) need to be obtained serially to follow brain growth and ventricular decompression. Once the ventricles have attained normal or subnormal size, this should be documented with a baseline CT or MRI scan. Further imaging studies of the head

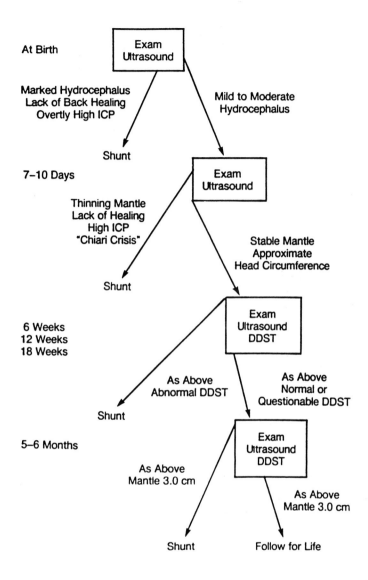

FIGURE 11. Algorithm of follow-up of children with spina bifida cystica and ventriculomegaly. (From Rekate, H. L., *Clin. Neurosurg.*, 32, 593, 1984. With permission.)

need to be obtained later only to assure proper functioning of the shunt or to document shunt failure and need not be performed at any routine interval.

If by 5 or 6 months, the ventricles have not decreased in size to the point that a 3.5-cm mantle can be assured, the function of the shunt must be tested operatively; if all parts are working, a lower pressure valve should be placed.

Implicit in the above discussion is the concept that normal flow of CSF is present in few children born with myelomeningocele. A decision not to shunt is certainly justifiable based on the risks of shunting; however, in the first 6 months of life, the unshunted child requires at least as compulsive a follow-up and assessment as does the child who has been shunted. When a doubt or question arises, the following adage is recommended: *When in doubt, shunt!*

REFERENCES

1. **Naidich, T. P., Pudlowski, R. M., Naidich, J. B., Gornish, M., and Rodriquez, F. J.,** Computed tomographic signs of the Chiari II malformation. I. Skull and dural partitions, *Radiology*, 134, 65, 1980.
2. **Lindseth, R. E.,** Orthopedic management of myelomeningocele, *BNI Q.*, 4(4), 26, 1988.
3. **Nulsen, F. E. and Spitz, E. B.,** Treatment of hydrocephalus by direct shunt from ventricle to jugular vein, *Surg. Forum*, 2, 399, 1952.
4. **Lorber, J.,** Results of treatment of myelomeningocele. An analysis of 524 unselected cases, with special reference to possible selection for treatment, *Dev. Med. Child Neurol.*, 13, 279, 1971.
5. **Lorber, J.,** Spina bifida cystica. Results of treatment of 270 consecutive cases with criteria for selection for the future, *Arch. Dis. Child*, 47, 854, 1972.
6. **Lonton, A. P., Barrington, N. A., and Lorber, J.,** Lacunar skull deformity related to intelligence in children with myelomeningocele and hydrocephalus, *Dev. Med. Child Neurol.*, 17(Suppl. 35), 58, 1975.
7. **McLone, D. G.,** Effect of complications on intellectual function in 173 children with myelomeningocele, *Child's Brain*, 5, A561, 1979.
8. **McLone, D. G., Killion, M., Yogev, R., and Sommers, M. W.,** Ventriculitis of mice and men, in *Concepts in Pediatric Neurosurgery*, Vol. 2, Epstein, F. and Raimondi, A., Eds., S. Karger, Basel, 1982, 112.
9. **Mapstone, T. B., Rekate, H. L., Nulsen, F. E., Dixon, M. S., Jr., Glaser, N., and Jaffe, M.,** Relationship of CSF shunting and IQ in children with myelomeningocele: a retrospective analysis, *Child's Brain*, 11, 112, 1984.
10. **Gross, R. H., Cox, A., Tatyrek, R., Pollay, M., and Barnes, W. A.,** Early management and decision making for the treatment of myelomeningocele, *Pediatrics*, 72, 450, 1983.
11. **Lyon, J.,** *Playing God in the Nursery*, W. W. Horton, New York, 1985, 59.
12. **Rekate, H. L.,** Early aggresive treatment of infants born with spina bifida: an ethical imperative, *BNI Q.*, 4(4), 2, 1988.
13. **Sharrard, W. J. W.,** The mechanism of paralytic deformity in spina bifida, *Dev. Med. Child Neurol.*, 4, 310, 1962.
14. **Sharrard, W. J.,** The segmental innervation of the lower limb muscles in man, *Ann. R. Coll. Surg. Engl.*, 35, 106, 1964.
15. **Sharrard, W. J. W., Zachary, R. B., Lorber, J., and Bruce, A. M.,** A controlled trial of immediate and delayed closure of spina bifida cystica, *Arch. Dis. Child*, 38, 18, 1963.
16. **Smyth, B. T., Piggot, J., Forsythe, W. I., and Merrett, J. D.,** A controlled trial of immediate and delayed closure of myelomeningocele, *J. Bone Joint Surg.*, 56B(2), 297, 1974.
17. **Charney, E. B., Weller, S. C., Sutton, L. N., Bruce, D. A., and Schut, L. B.,** Management of the newborn with myelomeningocele: time for a decision-making process, *Pediatrics*, 75(1), 58, 1985.

18. **Guthkelch, A. N.,** Studies in spina bifida cystica. II. When to repair the spinal defect, *J. Neurol. Neurosurg. Psychiat.*, 25, 137, 1962.

19. **Guthkelch, A. N.,** Thoughts on the surgical management of spina bifida cystica, *Acta Neurochir. (Wein)*, 13, 407, 1965.

20. **Guthkelch, A. N.,** Aspects of the surgical management of myelomeningocele: a review, *Dev. Med. Child Neurol.*, 28, 525, 1986.

21. **McLaurin, R. L.,** Myelomeningocele repair, *Contemp. Neurosurg.*, 6(17), 1, 1984.

22. **McLone, D. G.,** Technique for closure of myelomeningocele, *Child's Brain*, 6, 65, 1980.

23. **Habal, M. B. and Vries, J. K.,** Tension free closure of large meningomyelocele defects, *Surg. Neurol.*, 8, 177, 1977.

24. **Salasin, R. I. and Briggs, R. M.,** Closure of a large myelomeningocele. Case report, *Plast. Reconstr. Surg.*, 51, 464, 1973.

25. **Zook, E. G., Dzenitis, A. J., and Bennett, J. E.,** Repair of large myelomeningocele, *Arch. Surg.*, 98, 41, 1969.

26. **Desprez, J. D., Kiehn, C. L., and Eckstein, W.,** Closure of large meningomyelocele defects by composite skin-muscle flaps, *Plast. Reconstr. Surg.*, 47(3), 234, 1971.

27. **McDevitt, N. B., Gillespie, R. P., Woosley, R. E., Whitt, J. J., and Bevin, A. G.,** Closure of thoracic and lumbar dysgraphic defects using bilateral latissimuss dorsi myocutaneous flap transfer with extended gluteal fasciocutaneous flaps, *Child's Brain*, 9, 394, 1982.

28. **Moore, T. S., Dreyer, T. M., and Bevin, A. G.,** Closure of large spina bifida cystica defects with bilateral bipedicled musculocutaneous flaps, *Plast. Reconstr. Surg.*, 73, 288, 1984.

29. **Sharrad, W. J. W.,** Spinal osteotomy for congential kyphosis in myelomeningocele, *J. Bone Joint Surg.*, 50B, 466, 1968.

30. **Reigel, D. H.,** Kyphectomy and myelomeningocele repair, in *Modern Technique in Surgery*, Futura, Mount Kisco, NY, 1979, 1.

31. **Reigel, D. H.,** Indications for and technique of kyphectomy, in *Spina Bifida. A Multidisciplinary Approach*, McLaurin, R. L., Oppenheimer, S., Dias, L., and Kaplan, W. E. Eds., Praeger, New York, 1986, 140.

32. **Milhorat, T. H., Hammock, M. K., Fenstermacher, J. D., Rall, D. P., and Levin, V. A.,** Cerebrospinal fluid production by the choroid plexus and brain, *Science*, 173, 330, 1971.

33. **Rekate, H. and Olivero, W.,** Current concepts of CSF production and absorption, in *Hydrocephalus, Volume 3: Concepts in Neurosurgery*, Scott, R. M., Ed., Williams & Wilkins, Baltimore, 1989, 11.

34. **Rekate, H. L., Brodkey, J. A., Chizeck, H. J., El Sakka, W., and Ko, W. H.,** Ventricular volume regulation: a mathematical model and computer simulation, *Pediatr. Neurosci.*, 14, 77, 1988.

35. **Rekate, H. L., Williams, F., Chizeck, H. J., El Sakka, W., and Ko, W.,** The application of mathematical modeling to hydrocephalus research, in *Concepts in Pediatric Neurosurgery*, Vol. 8, Marlin, A. E., Ed., S. Karger, Basel, 1988, 1.

36. **Caldarelli, M., Di Rocco, C., amd Rossi, G. F.,** Lumbar subarachnoid infusion test in pediatric neurosurgery, *Dev. Med. Child Neurol.*, 21, 71, 1979.

37. **Sainte-Rose, C., LaCombe, J., Pierre-Kahn, A., Renier, D., and Hirsch, J.-F.,** Intracranial venous sinus hypertension: cause or donsequence of hydrocephalus in infants?, *J. Neurosurg.*, 60, 727, 1984.

38. **Steinbok, P., Hall, J., and Flodmark, O.,** Hydrocephalus and achondroplasia. The possible role of intracranial venous hypertension, *J. Neurosurg.*, 71, 42, 1989.

39. **Olivero, W. C., Rekate, H. L., Chizeck, H. J., Ko, W., and McCormick, J. M.,** Relationship between intracranial and sagittal sinus pressure in normal and hydrocephalic dogs, *Pediatr. Neurosci.*, 14, 196, 1988.

40. **Young, H. F., Nulsen, F. E., Weiss, M. H., and Thomas, P.,** The relationship of intelligence and verebral mantle in treated infantile hydrocephalus (IQ potential in hydrocephalic children), *Pediatrics*, 52, 38, 1973.

41. **Garbaciak, J. A., Jr.,** Obstetrical issues in spina bifida: perinatal management, prevention, and surgery, *BNI Q.*, 4(4), 9, 1988.

42. **Hubballah, M. Y. and Hoffman, H. J.,** Early repair of myelomeningocele and simultaneous insertion of ventriculoperitoneal shunt: technique and results, *Neurosurgery*, 20(1), 21, 1987.

43. **Laurence, K. M.,** Neurological and intellectual sequelae of hydrocephalus, *Arch. Neurol.*, 20, 73, 1969.

44. **Epstein, F.,** Diagnosis and management of arrested hydrocephalus, *Monogr. Neural. Sci.*, 8, 105, 1982.

45. **Epstein, F. J., Hochwald, G. M., Wald, A., and Ransohoff, J.,** Avoidance of shunt dependency on hydrocephalus, *Dev. Med. Child Neurol.*, 17(Suppl. 35), 71, 1975.

46. **Rekate, H. L., Nulsen, F. E., Mack, H. L., and Morrison, G.,** Establishing the diagnosis of shunt independence, *Monogr. Neural. Sci.*, 8, 223, 1982.

47. **Lewin, R.,** Is your brain really necessary?, *Science*, 210, 1232, 1980.

48. **Rekate, H. L.,** To shunt or not to shunt: hydrocephalus and dysraphism, *Clin. Neurosurg.*, 32, 593, 1985.

49. **Hall, P., Lindseth, R., Campbell, R., Kalsbeck, J. E., and Desousa, A.,** Scoliosis and hydrocephalus in myelocele patients. The effects of ventricular shunting, *J. Neurosurg.*, 50, 174, 1979.

50. **Jasper, P. L. and Merrill, R. E.,** Hydrocephalus and myelomeningocele: central nervous system infection, *Am. J. Dis. Child.*, 110, 652, 1965.

51. **O'Brien, M., Parent, A., and Davis, B.,** Management of ventricular shunt infections, *Child's Brain*, 5(3), 304, 1979.

52. **Venes, J. L.,** Control of shunt infection: report of 150 consecutive cases, *J. Neurosurg.*, 45, 311, 1976.

53. **Schoenbaum, S. C., Gardner, P., and Shillito, J.,** Infections of cerebrospinal fluid shunts: epidemiology, clinical manifestations, and therapy, *J. Infect. Dis.*, 131, 543, 1975.

54. **Klein, M.,** personal communication, 1980.

55. **Walker, M. L.,** personal communication, 1988.

Chapter 2

A CLINICAL VIEW OF THE EMBRYOLOGY
OF MYELOMENINGOCELE

Theodore J. Tarby

TABLE OF CONTENTS

I. INTRODUCTION

Despite its complexity, the human central nervous system (CNS) has its embryonic origin as a simple, tubular, ectodermal structure. Yet it is precisely this process, the establishment of the simple, tubular base for later elaboration, that goes awry in myelomeningocele. This relatively frequent congenital malformation of the CNS both provides us with clues to normal embryonic development and is better understood in terms of embryonic development.

In order to ultimately understand the structural abnormalities and the functional deficits that result from this developmental aberration, we need an embryologic foundation for both the normal and the aberrant structure. We must have a general appreciation of the embryologic events that lead to the development of the normal spinal cord. Then we can examine some of the theories that attempt to explain the abnormal structure of the myelomeningocele. It will become apparent that an understanding of the genesis of myelomeningocele requires a consideration of its virtually universal companion, the Chiari II (Arnold-Chiari) malformation. This, in turn, will require an appreciation of the normal development of the hindbrain and an examination of theories of the genesis of the Arnold-Chiari malformation. Finally, suggestions will be made as to the special variants of myelomeningocele that must be examined in order to make the next steps in our understanding of this common malformation complex.

II. EARLY EMBRYOGENESIS

The primordia of the human CNS are not evident from conception. A period of time must elapse before even the earliest recognizable precursor of the brain and spinal cord are apparent in the embryo. Yet it is clear that all of the information necessary for the development of the entire person, including the CNS, is present, if not appreciable, immediately after fertilization. Certain processes, events, or structures of early embryogenesis later appear to be important in neurogenesis. In order to better understand later nervous system development, we must briefly review early embryogenesis. We must also review the stages of embryonic development, the standard upon which the temporal sequence of human neurogenesis is based.

The development of the conceptus is divided into two major periods, embryogenesis and fetal development. Ovulation is the starting point of embryogenesis and fertilization its first event. Embryogenesis comprises the first 2 months of human gestation; the remaining 7 months are occupied with fetal development. The embryogenetic period has been extensively studied and the sequence of events in that period (partially) codified and placed in temporal sequence. The period of fetal development has not been so well described, thus events occurring during fetal development are commonly related to either the size of the fetus or to the gestational age. Since both menstrual and conceptual ages have been reported as gestational ages, there remains considerable confusion regarding the exact timing of events in fetal development.

A. Induction and the Organization of Embryogenesis

Embryologists have done a remarkable job of describing the changes in cellular, organic, and somatic morphology that occur during embryogenesis. They have made great strides in determining which cells or groups of cells control events at the various stages of embryonic development.[1,2] The mechanisms by which this control is exerted are largely obscure. In the absence of such understanding, these processes are referred to as induction. Thus, one structure, the organizer, is said to induce an event in another tissue or structure. Human organizers are not specifically known, rather they are inferred by analogy to experimentally identified organizers in other species.

In other vertebrate embryos, particularly in the avian embryo, structures known as the primitive streak, the notochord and the paraxial mesoderm, are important organizers of the early development of the CNS. These structures appear very early in embryogenesis. Once the primitive form of the CNS is established, further elaboration is felt to be controlled by other local organizers.

Following fertilization, several days of cell division are followed by cavitation of the resulting cellular mass to form the blastocyst. By day 4 or 5 of gestation, this blastocyst begins to implant itself onto the internal uterine surface. At this stage, there are two cavities within the blastocyst, the amniotic cavity and the yolk sac. Between these two cavities lies a bilaminar sheet within which will develop the embryo. The cell layer bathed in amniotic fluid is the ectoderm. The nervous system will develop from the neuroectoderm, a later specialization of the ectodermal layer of this simple embryo. The cell layer facing the yolk sac is the endoderm, the linings of the viscera will develop from this layer. Mesoderm will develop between these two layers. A major portion of somatic structure will develop from mesoderm.

B. Stages of Embryonic Development

Embryonic development in the human has been characterized as occurring in 23 stages,[3,4] frequently referred to as the Carnegie stages (Table 1). These stages are based on specific constellations of internal and external morphologic features present at a particular time in gestation. The 23 embryonic stages are internationally recognized. These developmental stages are not simply determined by embryonic length, but each stage has a length typical of that stage. Each stage of embryonic development lasts 1 to 6 d with the entire embryonic period encompassed in the first 2 months of gestation. The timing of the stages begins with the ovulation that results in conception; fertilization is thus the first stage and occurs on day 1 of gestation. The development of the nervous system has been related to these developmental stages.

The interrelationships between the events of nervous system development

TABLE 1
The Stages of Embryonic Development

Carnegie stage	Gestational age (d)[a]	Neuro-developmental events
1	0—1	Fertilization
2	1—4	
3	4—5	Blastocyst formation
4	6—9	Implantation
5	7—12	
6	13—15	Definition of disc axis
7	15—17	Localization of neural plate
8	17—19	Morphological neural plate
9	19—21	Neural groove, neural crest
10	22—23	Start of neural tube fusion
11	23—26	Closure of anterior neuropore
12	26—30	Closure of posterior neuropore Caudel cell mass present
13	28—32	Secondary neurulation begins with canalization
14	31—35	
15	33—38	
16	37—42	Retrogressive differentiation begins
17	40—44	
18	43—48	
19	45—51	
20	47—53	Canalization and union of the caudel elements with the neural tube is complete
21	48—54	
22	50—56	
23	52—60	Retrogressive differentiation continues until about day 80

Embryonic gestational age begins with ovulation; add 2 weeks for clinical gestational age.

and the developmental stages and in turn between the developmental stages and gestational age provide a basis for timing events in nervous system development. Establishing the time of occurrence of an insult or developmental deviation that results in a malformation is less precise. One can only be certain that an insult did not affect a particular developmental event if that event is complete before the insult. By contrast, a malformation may be caused by an insult occurring at the time the malformation becomes apparent or at any earlier time in gestation. Warkany[5] refers to the time after which a specific malformation cannot be produced as the termination period for that malformation. Volpe[6] has placed particular emphasis on this view of the genesis of CNS malformations. Such a perspective is important both clinically and scientifically, since it places at least a terminal limit on the time in gestation during which an insult could result in a specific malformation. It also emphasizes the importance of all prior development in setting the stage for any developmental event.

III. NORMAL NEUROGENESIS

A. Dorsal Induction

Dorsal induction refers to those processes which specify the ectodermal cells that will differentiate to become the CNS and to those interactions which result in the formation of the spinal cord and brain. The principal events of dorsal induction are those related to the early formation of the brain and those related to the formation of the majority of the spinal cord; these events comprise neurulation or primary neurulation. The formation of the caudal spinal cord is also a process of dorsal induction. Some authors refer to this process as secondary neurulation;[6] others consider the formation of the caudal spinal cord to be a postneurulation event.[7] Suffice it to say that the formation of the caudal spinal cord must be considered separately.

B. Specification

Nervous tissue is believed to be induced by an interaction between embryonic ectoderm and axial mesoderm or notochord derived from the primitive streak. It is not known how this specification of the nascent nervous system is accomplished and there is debate as to its timing. The best evidence to date suggests that neural specification occurs when the embryonic disk consists of only about 500 cells.[4] The resulting neuroectoderm includes the neural plate and the neural crest.

C. Primary Neurulation

The location of the neural plate has been determined as early as stage 7 or by 16 d gestation. By this stage, there are even zones identifiable that will become the sensory and the motor portions of the CNS (Figure 1). These zones are referred to as the alar and basal laminae, respectively. The neural plate itself can be identified morphologically by stage 8 or by 18 d gestation. It very rapidly begins to fold longitudinally to form the neural groove (Figure 2). As this folding proceeds into stage 9 (20 d gestation), the neural crest is formed at the lateral borders of the neural groove.

We have better knowledge of the mechanics of formation of the neural groove and subsequent neural tube than we do of the processes underlying induction.[8] It appears that the neuroectodermal cells within the neural plate elongate and constrict their dorsal (later apical or ventricular) surfaces. The

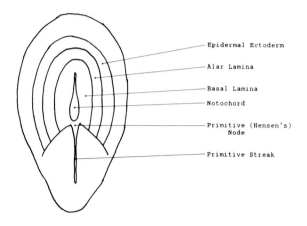

FIGURE 1. Schematic diagram of the neural plate.

elongation is produced by vertically oriented microtubules. Changes in the microtubules also result in a broadening of the ventral (later basal) surfaces of the cells. At the same time, contractile proteins in microfilaments oriented parallel to the apical ends of the cells cause these surfaces to constrict. The broadening of the basal surfaces and the constriction of the apical surfaces of the cells is restricted to the dimension orthogonal to the axis of the neural groove. The resulting deformation first produces the neural groove, then the neural tube.

By day 22 of gestation (stage 10), the apposed lips of the neural groove begin to fuse. Fusion begins in the region of the caudal rhombencephalon, that portion of the embryonic nervous system that will become the medulla. As in most tissues, cellular recognition and adhesion appear to be dependent on surface glycoproteins.[9] By the time that fusion of the neural tube is initiated, several discreet mounds of mesodermal cells have accumulated between the ectoderm and the endoderm. These are the first somites. The progression caudally of neurotube closure lags slightly behind the formation of additional somites. The first four somites are later incorporated into the occipital meso- dermal elements and no more rostral somites are formed. Nonetheless, rostral closure of the neural tube proceeds along with the caudally directed closure. As the neural tube forms, the adjacent somatic ectodermal layers also fuse, rees- tablishing the ectodermal (skin) surface. As this fusion occurs, groups of cells from the crest of each neural fold are pinched off from the neural tube. These neural crest cells differentiate into a variety of cell types, including the sensory neurons of the ganglia of spinal and cranial nerves, the postganglionic neurons of the autonomic nervous system, and the Schwann cells and satellite cells of the peripheral nervous system. The neural tube, on the other hand, develops into virtually the entire CNS. Its cavity becomes the ventricular system of the brain. At some unspecified point in this process, the rostral and caudal open-

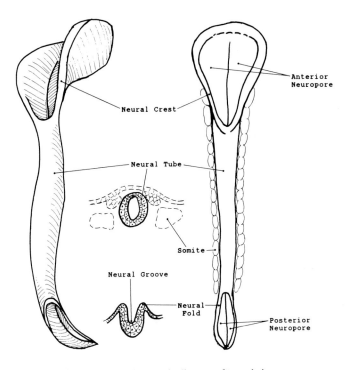

FIGURE 2. Schematic diagram of neurulation.

ings of the neural tube begin to be called the anterior (or rostral) and posterior (or caudal) neuropores, respectively.

During day 24 of gestation, in stage 11, the anterior neuropore closes. The processes and interactions underlying this event remain obscure. After the closure of the anterior neuropore, the cavity of the neural tube is open to the amniotic fluid only at the posterior neuropore. The posterior neuropore closes about 2 d later on day 26 of gestation, during stage 12. From this point onward, there is no communication between the central cavity of the neural tube (later the ventricular cavity/spinal central canal) and the embryonic body surface exposed to the amniotic fluid.

The exact site of posterior neuropore closure is variable but is generally somewhere in the upper lumbar spinal cord.[10] Posterior neuropore levels as high as T-11 and as low as the lumbosacral junction have been reported. This appears to be true variability around a most commonly quoted level of the L-1/L-2 interspace. The variable number of somites in the human embryo is the most likely cause of the variability in the location of the posterior neuropore. The more caudal segments of the lumbar and sacral spinal cord are formed by an entirely different process as discussed below.

D. Secondary Neurulation

Primary neurulation results in a closed neural tube with its caudal limit in

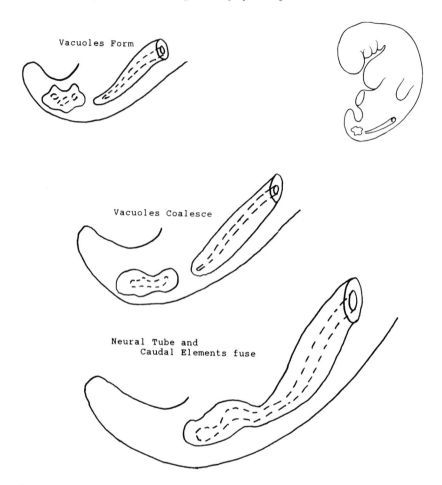

FIGURE 3. Schematic diagram of the junction between the closing neural tube and the caudal cell mass during secondary neurulation. Since both embryonic precursors are involved in myelomeningoceles, explanations of the genesis of myelomeningocele must encompass both.

what will be the lumbar (often upper lumbar) spinal cord. The formation of the remaining, most caudal, elements of the spinal cord and its coverings is related to the embryonic tail and its later disappearance (Figure 3).[6,11,12] The processes by which these most caudal elements are formed are known as canalization and retrogressive differentiation. Most authors seem to consider these processes as a completion of neurulation, though some consider the development of the caudal spinal cord to be a postneurulation event. The difference between these two views hinges on the observation that, as a consequence of neural tube formation, the neural tube becomes covered completely by somatic ectoderm or skin. By contrast, the more caudal elements of the spinal cord are formed beneath a covering of somatic ectoderm.

By the time of closure of the posterior neuropore during stage 12, an undifferentiated accumulation of cells is evident in the dorsal midline of the embryo, just caudal to the now closed neural tube. This cellular mass is known as the caudal eminence or the caudal cell mass. During stages 13 to 20, a remarkable and only partially elucidated series of events takes place. Early in this period, vacuoles appear in this cellular mass. These vacuoles are multiple and poorly organized. Each has the appearance of being a small central canal surrounded by an ependymal zone. Some vacuoles are larger than others and gradually there develops a clearly dominant central canal. This caudal cell mass and the primary neural tube make contact and continuity is established between the primary central canal and what will be the central canal of the caudal spinal cord. The primary neural tube and the multiple vacuoles in the caudal cell mass are each entirely closed before contact between the two elements is made. The adjacent walls of the caudal end of the primary neural tube and the rostral end of a vacuole in the caudal cell mass must break down to form the eventually continuous central canal. In addition, many of the vacuoles coalesce to extend the central canal caudally to a local dilation termed the terminal ventricle. This entire process has been named canalization.

When the process of canalization is maximal, there are 10 to 12 caudal vertebrae within the embryonic tail. Yet, even before canalization is complete (stage 20), tail regression has begun. Beginning in stage 16, caudal vertebrae fuse and regress. As the tail regresses there is a concurrent retrogressive differentiation of the caudal neural tube. This is most easily seen as a progressive ascent of the terminal ventricle. This retrogressive differentiation includes the excess growth of the lumbosacral spinal column as compared to the growth of the lumbosacral spinal cord. As the most caudal neural and meningeal elements atrophy, their degenerative remnant becomes the filum terminale. Despite the observations in humans summarized above, some authors contend that there is no extension of the neural tube caudal to the posterior neuropore.

E. Summary of Normal Neurulation

During week 3 of embryonic development, a longitudinal band of ectoderm thickens to form the neural plate. Shortly thereafter, the neural plate begins to fold inward, forming a longitudinal neural groove in the midline flanked by a parallel neural fold on each side. The neural groove deepens, and the neural folds approach each other in the dorsal midline. At the end of week 3 the two folds begin to fuse, thus forming the neural tube and reestablishing the ectodermal (skin) surface. As this fusion occurs, groups of cells from the crest of each neural fold are pinched off from the neural tube. These neural crest cells develop into a variety of cell types, including the sensory neurons of the ganglia of spinal and cranial nerves, the postganglionic neurons of the autonomic nervous system, and the Schwann cells and satellite cells of the peripheral nervous system. The neural tube, on the other hand, develops into virtually the entire CNS; its cavity becomes the ventricular system of the brain.

The area of fusion of the two neural folds, which begins in the cervical region of the future spinal cord, rapidly expands rostrally (toward the future brain) and caudally (toward the sacral end of the future spinal cord). The anterior (rostral) neuropore, the opening at the rostral end of the neural tube, closes completely in the middle of week 4; the posterior (caudal) neuropore closes about 2 d later. As each successive bit of neural tube is formed by the progressive fusion of the neural folds, it becomes separated from the overlying ectoderm, and mesodermal elements are interposed between somatic ectoderm and neural tube.

A small but important portion of the caudal neural plate forms the lumbosacral neural tube and spinal cord by a different mechanism: canalization and retrogressive differentiation.

IV. THE CHIARI II MALFORMATION

All or virtually all patients born with myelomeningocele also have a malformation of the hindbrain and upper cervical spinal cord. This malformation has had a number of eponyms applied to it, most of which are difficult to justify historically.[13,14] The two most commonly used eponyms are the Chiari II malformation and the Arnold-Chiari malformation. Arnold's contribution to the description and understanding of this hindbrain malformation was minimal. He did, however, have two proteges who, in attributing priority to him, confused the literature. To make matters worse, at least from an attributional standpoint, Cleland[15] described this malformation 8 years before Chiari.

Chiari originally described three malformations of the cerebellum which were accompanied by hydrocephalus. The Chiari II malformation is described below. In the Chiari I malformation, the cerebellar tonsils protrude caudally through the foramen magnum and often into the spinal canal. Most authors agree that Chiari did not describe any caudal displacement of the brain stem in this first and least severe malformation. It has been suggested that the Chiari I malformation exists as two distinct entities, one as described above and the second which includes herniation of both the cerebellar tonsils and the brain stem (but not the vermis) through the foramen magnum.[16,17] The Chiari III malformation involves herniation of the brain stem caudally into a bifid cervical spinal canal. The cerebellum is contained in a cervical encephalocele. Interestingly, this severe malformation is only occasionally accompanied by a caudal myelomeningocele. A Chiari IV malformation involving cerebellar aplasia has been described, but is no longer felt to relate to this sequence of malformations. Indeed, the three original Chiari malformations may have three different embryologic origins.

The Chiari II malformation is found in all (or virtually all) patients with myelomeningocele and only very rarely in other patients.[16-23] It consists of displacement of the inferior cerebellar vermis, caudal fourth ventricle, and medulla oblongata into the cervical spinal canal. Besides these defining characteristics, a large number of associated findings, some developmental, some secondary, may be present. In rare individuals, often with a small and very low myelomeningocele, the cardinal features of the Chiari II malformation may be undetectable (at least in life) while its presence is signaled by a host of associated features.

In the Chiari II malformation, the vermis appears atrophic, but is otherwise not dysplastic. The cerebellar hemispheres are small as is the entire posterior fossa. The tentorium cerebelli, which is vertically oriented, arises from a caudally displaced peripheral attachment. This in turn results in a low placed torcula. The venous sinuses are similarly low set and appear large. The tentorial incisure is enlarged and the falx is often hypoplastic.

The pons, medulla, and cervicomedullary junction are all displaced caudally as are the basilar and vertebral arteries. There is frequently a distortion of the medulla referred to as a medullary kink. The upper segments of the cervical spinal cord are compressed; there may be hydromyelia or syringomyelia. There is stretching of the lower cranial nerves and the upper cervical roots course rostrally. There is distortion of the midbrain referred to as tectal beaking. The cerebral aqueduct may be stenotic or forked.

The malformation is frequently accompanied by hydrocephalus. The hydrocephalus may be evident during the second trimester and massive at birth or may be absent at birth only to develop during the first 6 months of life. While it is tempting to attribute the hydrocephalus to the abnormalities found in the cerebral aqueduct, the two are not always associated. Hydrocephalus may be present when the aqueduct is demonstrably patent. Polymicrogyria, cortical heterotopias and an enlarged massa intermedia are commonly present.

The skull and cervical spine of the patient with the Chiari II malformation are frequently abnormal. The posterior fossa is small, the foramen magnum is enlarged. Craniolacunae are frequently present and the petrous bones appear to be scalloped. Platybasia may be evident. The spinal canal may be widened in the upper cervical region.

V. THEORIES OF THE EMBRYOGENESIS OF MYELOMENINGOCELE AND OF THE CHIARI II MALFORMATION

A. Some Statistics

Spina bifida cystica, including but not limited to myelomeningocele, may occur at any vertebral level. Published series[24] of cases may be regrouped into three categories (Table 2): (1) isolated cervical or thoracic spina bifida cystica; (2) spina bifida cystica that includes the lumbar spinal cord, either alone or in combination with either thoracic or sacral segments or both; and (3) isolated sacral spina bifida cystica. Of these, defects that involve the lumbar cord account for 78% of the cases, while sacral defects account for an additional 10% of cases and isolated cervical and thoracic defects combined for 11% of

TABLE 2
Distribution of Spina Bifida Cystica[a]

Defect level	No.	%
Cervical		38	4.1
Thoracic		63	6.8
Isolated			10.9
Thoracolumbar	103	11.1
Thoracolumbosacral	23	2.5
Lumbar	360	39.0
Lumbosacral	231	25.0
Posterior neuropore involved			77.6
Sacral		93	10.1
Caudal cell mass only			10.1
Thoracolumbosacral	23	2.5
Lumbosacral	231	25.0
Sacral		93	10.1
Caudal cell mass involved			37.6
Other/unspecified	10	1.1

[a] Modified from a paper by Welch and Winston.[24]

the tabulated cases. Sacral and lumbosacral defects combined represented 35% of these cases.

Meningoceles, myelocystoceles, and syringomyeloceles were acknowledged to be rare and to occur at any spinal cord level. These lesions are likely to be disproportionately represented in the cervical and thoracic cases. Thus, approximately 80% of the myelomeningoceles involve the region of posterior neural tube closure, but about 35% include segments derived from the caudal cell mass. Since the usual site of posterior neural tube closure is in the upper lumbar cord, considerably more than 10% of myelomeningoceles can be expected to develop wholly in segments derived from the caudal cell mass. In addition, the existence of thoracolumbar and lumbar myelomeningoceles suggests that the caudal cell mass may differentiate reasonably normally despite a more superior defect. The preservation of the anal wink in such patients has led to a similar conclusion on clinical grounds.[25] Any comprehensive description of the embryogenesis of myelomeningocele must encompass these observations.

B. General Observations

The embryogenesis of the dysraphic states has been and is the subject of considerable speculation and debate.[6,7,10-16,20,23,26-37] Our knowledge and understanding of these aberrant processes is incomplete. That does not seriously inhibit the development of hypotheses purporting to explain these complex events. Since it is the testing of hypotheses that leads to knowledge, it is important to recognize the deficiencies of the various hypotheses so that the questions so generated may someday lead to understanding.

It may well be that no single embryogenic mechanism is adequate to explain all of the rich variety of neural tube defect. That is certainly the case if both open and closed defects are included. It is probably true as well if only the most common defect, the open myelomeningocele is considered. Since the caudal spinal cord apparently forms underneath an ectodermal (skin) layer, observations which appear to support one mechanism rostrally may find conflict caudally. Myelomeningoceles involving the posterior neuropore may have one embryogenic mechanism, while those derived from the caudal cell mass, another. In each case, the degree of association of the dysraphic condition with the Chiari II malformation will have to be considered.

There have been numerous classifications of the theories regarding the embryogenesis of the myelomeningocele. The outline presented here is synthetic and meant to lead to two recent proposals that appear to be mutually exclusive. In evaluating theories of the embryogenesis of myelomeningocele, two major issues need to be addressed. The first is whether the mechanism proposed results in a failure of neural tube closure or in a reopening of the closed neural tube. Second, it is important to know whether the Chiari II malformation is to be held responsible for or a consequence of the process that leads to the myelomeningocele.

C. Myelomeningocele as a Failure of Neurulation

Experimental evidence that myelomeningocele can result from failure of the posterior neural tube to undergo normal closure during week 4 of gestation appears compelling. The termination period for such a myelomeningocele is probably no later than 26 d of gestation. This time in week 4 of gestation marks the end of normal neural tube closure. Mechanisms that involve a failure of neural tube closure would be expected to be complete by this time. Agents that impair normal neural tube closure produce neural tube defects, including myelomeningocele, when administered to animals.

When animals genetically predisposed to the development of neural tube defects are examined, myelomeningocele is seen to result from a failure of neural tube closure. Both the curly-tail mouse[35] and the delayed splotch mouse[34] display this feature. In the curly-tail mouse, Seller and Adinolfi[35] were unable to find any example of a normally closed neural tube that subsequently developed myelomeningocele.

Pathologic examination of aborted human embryos has revealed myeloschisis and myelomeningocele at embryological stages prior to, or immediately following, completion of neural tube closure. Osaka et al.[36] demonstrated thoracolumbar myeloschisis in a 27 d embryo. Lemire et al.[37] reported caudal myeloschisis or lumbosacral spina bifida cystica in a 5-mm human embryo.

This embryo was noted to be at horizon (stage) XIV, indicating that the lesion had occurred before closure of the neural tube. These lesions occurred long before the appearance of the choroid plexus (approximately 43 d).

An overgrowth of neuroectoderm is frequently seen in these embryos. It is not clear whether this overgrowth is causative or a consequence of the dysraphic condition. At present, the bulk of evidence suggests that most myelomeningoceles result from an impairment in primary neural tube closure. In these theories, the genesis of the Chiari II malformation is secondary, requiring specific explanation.

These studies uniformly fail to address the issue of the spinal cord defect that extends into that portion of the spinal cord that develops from the caudal cell mass. Sacral, and some lumbosacral, myelomeningoceles are expected to be derived wholly from the caudal cell mass. An alternative mechanism is required in these instances.

D. Myelomeningocele as a Sequela of Hydrocephalus

An alternative to the theory of abnormal neural tube closure holds that the tube closes normally, but later is ruptured by abnormal hydrodynamic forces, i.e., hydrocephalus. Gardner et al.[29] extended this concept to an alternative explanation for the origin not only of the myelomeningocele and Chiari II malformation, but also for the Dandy-Walker malformation and for the cerebral accompaniments of the Chiari II malformation.

Gardner proposed that the neural tube closes but is reopened by an abnormal hydrodynamic state. This abnormal hydrodynamic state is said to be caused by a persistent impermeability of the roof of the fourth ventricle that impairs cerebrospinal fluid (CSF) outflow. The pulsating choroid plexus results in an abnormal pulsating hydrodynamic state that distends the central canal of the developing spinal cord. This abnormally distended state is termed hydrocephalomyelia. A variety of specific conditions are held then to result in a spectrum of CNS malformations. In the case of myelomeningocele, hydrocephalomyelia is held eventually to rupture the caudal neural tube.

Weed's description of the development of the fourth ventricle is important in the genesis of this theory.[38] In this description, there is a phase in the development of the fourth ventricle in which the roof is contended to be impermeable to CSF. Brocklehurst[14] has presented evidence that the perforation of the rhombencephalic roof is a developmental process rather than mechanistic rupture occasioned by increased pressure. Pathologic studies of early embryos with dysraphic states have not provided histological evidence for an abnormal roof to the fourth ventricle nor for rupture of the neural tube.

This theory, moreover, is inconsistent with reports demonstrating that myeloschisis occurs in human embryos before the formation of the choroid plexus.[36,37] It has been contended that osmotic pressure produced by the proteinaceous fluid is sufficient to distend and rupture the primitive neural tube. Early embryos displaying myeloschisis have not been noted to have cerebral hydrocephalus. In addition, it is difficult to accept this explanation for extensive lesions approaching or including craniorachischisis. Such lesions would be expected to have dissipated the inciting abnormal pressure long before the entire lesion could be produced.

As noted above, animal studies have shown that once a neural tube has closed, there is no subsequent development of myelomeningocele. Thus, at the present time, there is little evidence to support the notion that myelomeningocele is caused by secondary rupture of the closed neural tube. The deficiencies in accounting for the genesis of the myelomeningocele have resulted in a tendency to dismiss out of hand all aspects of the hydrocephalus theory. Pressure relationships are still held by some to be important in the genesis of the Chiari II malformation. In addition, hydrocephalus is certainly important in exacerbating the clinical features of the Chiari II malformation.

E. Myelomeningocele Secondary to Neuroschisis

In contrast to the theories that postulate abnormal pressure relationships within the embryonic central canal, the theory of neuroschisis proposed by Padget[39] suggests that an abnormal cleft is formed in the closed neural tube. This cleft is thought to weaken the developing neural tube allowing rupture and escape of CSF. The proteinaceous fluid that escapes through the defect collects in the mesoderm, elevating the overlying cutaneous ectoderm. This embryologic entity has been termed a neuroschistic bleb. This mechanism, combined with secondary factors, such as the time and location of the neuroschistic injury is postulated as explaining the genesis of a variety of neural tube defects.

The neuroschistic bleb may heal completely or it may rupture to the cutaneous surface, creating an open spinal lesion. The opening might be lined with cutaneous ectoderm as in a congenital dermal sinus tract. Alternatively, it could result in the fusion of the cutaneous ectoderm with the neuroectoderm. This would appear as a defect that had never closed. Some of the same arguments presented above may be directed against this form of secondary rupture of the closed neural tube. Injury of this type, however, may be important in specific experimental models of neural tube dysgenesis without establishing their role in the human condition.[40]

While this mechanism may not pertain to spinal defects that involve the posterior neuropore, it may well be the mechanism or a portion of the mechanism underlying defects in those spinal segments derived from the caudal cell mass.

F. Myelomeningocele Secondary to Vascular Abnormalities

Stevenson et al.[33] have shown that the arterial supply to the region of a neural tube defect is abnormal. The arterial supply to the neural folds is established before the closure of the neural tube. These observations have led to the hypothesis that neural tube defects are produced by a delay in establishing blood flow or an aberration in blood supply to developing neural tissue. The vascular abnormalities are considered to be primary malformations that lead to neural tube defects rather than secondary disturbances that result from the nervous system abnormality. These observations have also been suggested to support the failure of closure mechanism rather than the reopening hypotheses.

No explanation of the relationship of the Chiari II malformation to the abnormal vasculature was provided. Other studies have suggested that meso-dermal injury or disruption is the primary event in neural tube defects.[30]

G. The Traction Theory for the Chiari II Malformation

It has been suggested that the fixation of the spinal cord to the skin at the site of a myelomeningocele prevents upward migration of the spinal cord during development and results in the Chiari II malformation. According to this theory, the brain stem and cerebellum are elongated and pulled down into the spinal canal as the vertebral column elongates. Clinical, pathologic, and experimental objections to this theory are overwhelming.[6,23,32,34] The traction theory for the genesis of the Chiari II malformation is generally considered to be discredited.

H. Neuroectodermal-Mesodermal Dyssynchrony as a Cause of the Chiari II Malformation

Jennings et al.[31] examined a 130-d female human fetus with the Chiari II malformation and thoracolumbar myeloschisis. The fetus was 173 mm in crown-rump length. They observed that reports based on gestational specimens are rare, though the essential features of the Chiari II malformation have been identified as early as 49 to 50 mm crown-rump length in the human. The lack of such specimens was felt to compound the problem of distinguishing developmental anomalies from secondary deformations.

Their specimen exhibited obvious hydrocephalus and a myeloschisis that extended from T6 caudally. The cerebral aqueduct was distended. The fourth ventricle was small. The cerebellum was represented only by an incipient left hemisphere extending laterally from a midline cerebellar ridge. There was no obvious mechanical cause for the hydrocephalus. Cranial concomitants of the Chiari II malformation were present. These included a small posterior fossa and an inferiorly attached tentorium cerebelli. The base of the skull appeared to be normal. The vertebral bodies from C4 to C7 were hypoplastic and were paralleled by a hypoplastic appearance to the spinal cord. The spine below T6 was fused into a single mass. Interestingly, the spinal ganglia adjacent to the myeloschisis retained their segmental organization.

The lower pons and medulla were displaced caudally into the spinal canal. A variable degree of displacement and dysgenesis were seen, with the most severe abnormalities at the level of the rhombencephalon, then in the lower cervical cord, and finally in the myeloschisis itself. Intervening segments of the spinal cord were less significantly displaced and more normal in appearance.

The authors suggest that the development of the caudal rhombencephalon and the establishment of the cervicomedullary junction at the level of the foramen magnum are the critical events around which the pathogenesis of the Chiari II malformation occurs. They hypothesize that the initiating event in the development of the Chiari II malformation is the caudal displacement of the site of initial fusion of the neural folds. This displaces the brain cord transition zone caudally relative to the adjacent mesoderm. Thus, the hindbrain would develop within the spinal canal and neither be pushed nor pulled into it. The disorganization within the medulla is seen as supporting this hypothesis and implying an early insult. The essential error in the genesis of the Chiari II malformation is thus held to be neuroectodermal-mesodermal dyssynchrony.

The dyssynchrony would cause displacement, both spatially and temporally, of a putative gradient that induces caudal neural fold fusion. This in turn would result in permanent myeloschisis that persists despite the later development of somites and neural crest derivatives adjacent to the zone of myeloschisis. The authors suggest that their hypothesis explains the close association of thoracolumbar myeloschisis with the Chiari II malformation. The issue of extension of the myeloschisis into the segments derived from the caudal cell mass is not considered, nor is the preservation of those segments in some cases of thoracolumbar or lumbar myelomeningocele.

I. Ventricular Collapse as a Cause of the Chiari II Malformation

McLone and Knepper[34] have recently presented a unified theory of the cause of the Chiari II malformation. Their theory is based on studies of the genetic model of abnormal neurulation, the delayed Splotch (Spd/Spd) mouse embryo. Mice homozygous for this autosomal recessive gene develop caudal neural tube defects. The neurulation defect is held to be an *a priori* feature of the development of the Chiari II malformation. Abnormalities in the complex carbohydrates on the cell surface and within the extracellular matrix are believed to disrupt signals required for cellular differentiation and maturation. This disruption leads to a sacral neurulation defect.

The neurulation defect was seen to result in a failure of the normal apposition of the ventral walls of the caudal neurotube. This in turn allowed a decompression (or a failure to maintain the distention) of the primitive cranial ventricular system. This failure of the normal apposition is accompanied by further evidence of abnormalities in the composition of the complex carbohydrates at cell surfaces in the developing neural tube.

The inability to maintain distension of the primitive ventricular system is said to result in the development of a small posterior fossa. This is said to occur despite the transient nature of the ventral occlusion of the neural tube. It is not known whether the failure of normal apposition represents an inadequacy of apposition or an abnormality of its timing. The development of the cerebellum and brain stem occur within the fixed and inadequate volume of the posterior fossa. Subsequent to these events, the brain stem moves caudally, coming to rest below the foramen magnum. Since the volume of the posterior fossa is fixed by endochondral bone formation, further growth and development of posterior fossa structures results in upward herniation accompanied by a dysplastic tentorium and an enlarged incisure.

The inability to maintain distension of the primitive ventricular system is also seen to result in the forebrain concomitants of the Chiari II malformation. Inadequate distension of the third ventricle is seen to result in an enlarged massa intermedia. In experimental animals, draining the telencephalic ventricles resulted in disorganization of the cerebral cortex.[41] Abnormalities of both endochondral (shortened clivus) and membranous (lückenschädel) bone formation are believed to be a consequence of inadequate distension of the primitive ventricular system.

The final step in the developmental sequence putatively set in process by the caudal defect is hydrocephalus. The causes of the hydrocephalus are multiple, but are believed to be secondary to mistimed steps in the development of the ventricular system.

VI. CONCLUSIONS

There is now compelling evidence that posterior neural tube closure is defective in a majority of myelomeningoceles. Open defects that involve those spinal cord segments derived from the caudal cell mass require a different mechanism for their development. This is a sizable portion of human cases of myelomeningocele, perhaps 25 to 33% of all tabulated cases. A reopening mechanism must operate in these cases since the caudal cell mass develops beneath a cutaneous ectodermal covering.

Two recent publications have served to reopen the controversy over the genesis of the Chiari II malformation and its relation to the myelomeningocele. In one, abnormal neurulation is seen to result in the decompression of the primitive ventricular system. This primary event is followed by a sequence of developmental aberrations leading ultimately to the full spectrum of abnormalities seen in the Chiari II malformation. In the other, the primary event is believed to be the caudal displacement of the site of initial fusion of the neural folds. This neuroectodermal-mesodermal dyssynchrony in turn results in the posterior displacement of the cervico-medullary junction and myeloschisis. Both are logical and internally consisten; thus they form fertile ground for renewed investigation into their conclusions.

Careful analysis of rare events such as isolated or multiple zones of myeloschisis, Chiari II malformations without myelomeningocele, or even myelomeningocele without Chiari II malformation, may provide the next steps in our understanding of the genesis of this common and debilitating complex.

REFERENCES

1. **Kallen, B.,** Errors in the differentiation of the central nervous system, in *Handbook of Clinical Neurology, Vol. 6(50): Malformations,* Myrianthopoulos, N. C., Ed., Elsevier, Amsterdam, 1987, chap. 2.

2. **Purves, D. and Lichtman, J. W.,** *Principles of Neural Development,* Sinauer Associates, Sunderland, MA, 1985, chap. 3.

3. **Lemire, R. J., Loeser, J. D., Leech, R. W., and Alvord, E. C., Jr.,** *Normal and Abnormal Development of the Human Nervous System,* Harper & Row, Hagerstown, MD, 1975, chap. 1.

4. **O'Rahilly, R and Muller, F.,** The developmental anatomy and histology of the human central nervous system, in *Handbook of Clinical Neurology, Vol. 6(50): Malformations,* Myrianthopoulos, N. C., Ed., Elsevier, Amsterdam, 1987, chap. 1.

5. **Warkany, J.,** *Congenital Malformations,* Year Book Medical Publishers, Chicago, 1971, chap. 1.

6. **Volpe, J. J.,** *Neurology of the Newborn,* 2nd ed., W. B. Saunders, Philadelphia, 1987, chap. 1.

7. **Lemire, R. J.,** Neural tube defects, *JAMA,* 259, 558, 1988.

8. **Karfunkel, P.,** The mechanisms of neural tube formation, *Int. Rev. Cytol.,* 38, 245, 1974.

9. **McClone, D. G., Suwa, J., Collins, J. A., Poznanski, S., and Knepper, P. A.,** Neurulation: biochemical and morphological studies on primary and secondary neural tube defects, *Concept. Pediatr. Neurosurg.,* 4, 15, 1983.

10. **Lemire, R. J., Loeser, J. D., Leech, R. W., and Alvord, E. C., Jr.,** *Normal and Abnormal Development of the Human Nervous System,* Harper & Row, Hagerstown, MD, 1975, chap. 4.

11. **Lemire, R. J., Loeser, J. D., Leech, R. W., and Alvord, E. C., Jr.,** *Normal and Abnormal Development of the Human Nervous System,* Harper & Row, Hagerstown, MD, 1975, chap. 5.

12. **French, B. N.,** The embryology of spinal dysraphism, *Clin. Neurosurg.,* 30, 295, 1983.

13. **Carmel, P. W.,** The Arnold-Chiari malformation, in *Pediatric Neurosurgery: Surgery of the Developing Nervous System,* Grune & Stratton, New York, 1982, chap. 4.

14. **Brocklehurst, G.,** The pathogenesis of spina bifida: a study of the relationship between observation, hypothesis and surgical incentive, *Develop. Med. Child Neurol.,* 13, 147, 1971.

15. **Cleland, J.,** Contribution to the study of spina bifida, encephalocele, and anencephalus, *J. Anat. Physiol.,* 17, 257, 1883.

16. **Roessmann, U.,** The embryology and neuropathology of congenital malformations, *Clin. Neurosurg.,* 30, 157, 1983.

17. **Friede, R. L. and Roessmann, U.,** Chronic tonsillar herniation, *Acta Neuropathol. (Berlin),* 34, 219, 1976.

18. **Peach, B.,** Arnold-Chiari malformation with normal spine, *Arch. Neurol.,* 10, 497, 1964.

19. **Emery, J. L. and MacKenzie, N.,** Medullo-cervical dislocation deformity (Chiari II deformity) related to neurospinal dysraphism (meningomyelocele), *Brain,* 96, 155, 1973.

20. **Salam, M. Z. and Adams, R. D.,** The Arnold-Chiari malformation, in *Handbook of Clinical Neurology, Vol. 32, Congenital Malformations of the Spine and Spinal Cord,* Vinken, P. J. and Bruyn, G. W., Eds., North-Holland, Amsterdam, 1978, chap. 2.

21. **Naidich, T. P., Harwood-Nash, D. C., and McLone, D. G.,** Radiology of spinal dysraphism, *Clin. Neurosurg.,* 30, 341, 1983.

22. **Gilbert, J. N., Jones, K. L., Rorke, L. B., Chernoff, G. F., and James, H. E.,** Central nervous system anomalies associated with meningomyelocele, hydrocephalus, and the Arnold-Chiari malformation: reappraisal of theories regarding the pathogenesis of posterior neural tube closure defects, *Neurosurgery,* 18, 559, 1986.

23. **Bamberger-Bozo, C.,** The Chiari II malformation, in *Handbook of Clinical Neurology, Vol. 6(50): Malformations,* Myrianthopoulos, N. C., Ed., Elsevier, Amsterdam, 1987, chap. 23.

24. **Welch, K. and Winston, K. R.,** Spina bifida, in *Handbook of Clinical Neurology, Vol. 6(50): Malformations,* Myrianthopoulos, N. C., Ed., Elsevier, Amsterdam, 1987, chap. 29.

25. **Guthkelch, A. N.,** Studies in spina bifida cystica. V.: Anomalous reflexes in congenital spinal palsy, *Develop. Med. Child Neurol.,* 6, 264, 1964.

26. **Barry, A., Patten, B. M., and Stewart, B. H.,** Possible factors in the development of the Arnold-Chiari malformation, *J. Neurosurg.,* 14, 285, 1957.

27. **Peach, B.,** The Arnold-Chiari malformation: morphogenesis, *Arch. Neurol.,* 12, 527, 1965.

28. **van Hoytema, G. J. and van den Berg, R.,** Embryological studies of the posterior fossa in connection with Arnold-Chiari malformation, *Develop. Med. Child Neurol.,* Suppl. 11, 61, 1966.

29. **Gardner, E., O'Rahilly, R., and Prolo, D.,** The Dandy-Walker and Arnold-Chiari malformations, *Arch. Neurol.,* 32, 393, 1975.

30. **Marin-Padilla, M.,** Clinical and experimental rachischisis, in *Handbook of Clinical Neurology,* Vol. 32, *Congenital Malformations of the Spine and Spinal Cord,* Vinken, P. J. and Bruyn, G. W., Eds., North-Holland, Amsterdam, 1978, chap. 6.

31. **Jennings, M. T., Clarren, S. K., Kokich, V. G., and Alvord, E. C., Jr.,** Neuroanatomic examination of spina bifida aperta and the Arnold-Chiari malformation in a 130-day human fetus, *J. Neurol. Sci.,* 54, 325, 1982.

32. **Noetzel, M. J. and Volpe, J. J.,** Neural tube defects, in *Handbook of the Spinal Cord,* Vol. 4, Davidoff, R. A., Ed., Marcel Dekker, New York, 1987, chap. 8.

33. **Stevenson, R. E., Kelly, J. C., Aylsworth, A. S., and Phelan, M. C.,** Vascular basis for neural tube defects: a hypothesis, *Pediatrics,* 80, 102, 1987.

34. **McLone, D. G. and Knepper, P. A.,** The cause of the Chiari II malformation: a unified theory, *Pediatr. Neurosci.,* 15, 1, 1989.

35. **Seller, M. J. and Adinolfi, M.,** The curly-tail mouse: an experimental model for human neural tube defects, *Life Sci.,* 29, 1607, 1981.

36. **Osaka, K., Matsumoto, S., and Tanimura, T.,** Myelomeningocele in early human embryos, *Child's Brain,* 4, 347, 1978.

37. **Lemire, R. J.,** Caudal myeloschisis (lumbro-sacral spina bifida cystica) in a five millimeter (Horizon XIV) human embryo, *Anat. Rec.,* 152, 9, 1965.

38. **Weed, L. H.,** The development if the cerebrospinal spaces in pig and man, *Contrib. Embryol. Carnegie Inst.,* 5, 1, 1917.

39. **Padget, D. H.,** Spina bifida and embryonic neuroschisis, *Johns Hopkins Med. J.,* 128, 233, 1968.

40. **Katz, M. J.,** CNS effects of mechanically produced spina bifida, *Develop. Med. Child Neurol.,* 26, 617, 1984.

41. **Coulombre, A. J. and Coulombre, J. L.,** The role of mechanical factors in brain morphogenesis, *Anat. Rec.,* 130, 289, 1958.

Chapter 3

PEDIATRIC MANAGEMENT OF CHILDREN WITH MYELODYSPLASIA

Morris S. Dixon, Jr. and Harold L. Rekate

TABLE OF CONTENTS

In the treatment of children with myelodysplasia, as in the case of many congenital anomalies, the role of the pediatrician as the one physician member of the multidisciplinary care team who sees the child as a whole person is both crucial and central. In addition to the various neurosurgical, orthopedic, and urologic crises inevitably encountered, both the child and his or her family will have to handle the hard job of growing up with multiple disabilities. As the trustee of the goals of the child from a medical perspective, it is the pediatrician who insures that these goals are understood by all of the child's caretakers and that no one is working at cross purposes. The emphasis on well child care, so important in the problem-oriented medical recordkeeping in pediatrics, is easy to forget.

In the midst of the care so often required by children with conditions as difficult as spina bifida, it is easy to overlook or postpone issues such as bowel management, inspection of anesthetic skin areas, and weight control when the child cannot expend calories by increased activities of the lower extremities that rarely occur and are largely managed with minimal guidance in other populations of children.

Two pediatricians are needed to insure the well-being of the child with spina bifida. This discussion emphasizes the pediatric member of the multidisciplinary team who is essential to the optimal management of the child. The other pediatrician is the primary care pediatrician in the community who is taking care of the pediatric needs of the child and probably the siblings. The community pediatrician must receive continuous updates on the medical care of the child from the team and, as much as possible, remain a part of the team.

I. INITIAL ASSESSMENT AND MANAGEMENT

An article published in 1982[1] suggested that the incidence of myelodysplasia is decreasing, at least in the U.S. Other studies have also confirmed the declining incidence in many other countries.[2,3] Despite these statistics, myelodysplasia is still one of the most common serious congenital abnormalities.[4] However, these statistics are not important to the parents of a newborn with myelodysplasia who were expecting a normal infant and are now confronted with a child with multiple abnormalities.

With obvious deformities so apparent at the time of birth, the obstetrician is the first individual to become involved with the care of the mother and infant. The diagnosis is readily made by gross inspection. Generally, the obstetrician tells the mother the baby has an abnormality and requests pediatric consultation to assist with the immediate management of the infant. Unless the baby is born in an institution that cares for many children with myelodysplasia, the infant should be transferred to a tertiary care hospital for further assessment and treatment. During the first contact with the parents, the obstetrician and pediatrician should be cautious about the prognosis but should assure the parents that definitive information will be forthcoming in a few hours. The

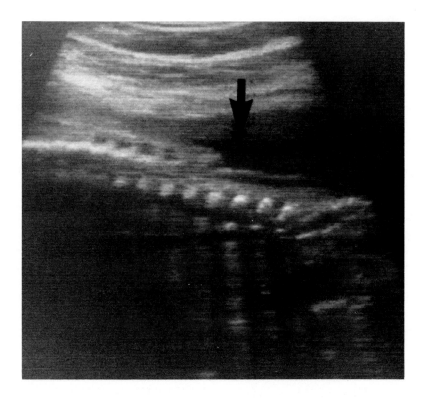

FIGURE 1. Ultrasound examination of preterm infant with spina bifida evident.

parents will be extremely sensitive and will remember this first contact for years. If, as is so often the case, the pediatrician gives a dismal prognosis, the parents will be unforgiving. It also makes it more difficult for the specialists to undo misconceptions later.

With the increasing availability and utilization of prenatal screening procedures, such as maternal serum α-fetoprotein (AFP) analysis, amniocentesis, and uterine ultrasound procedures, the number of prenatally diagnosed cases of spina bifida is increasing (Figure 1). When the diagnosis of spina bifida is made in the fetus, the parents should be seen by a pediatrician or pediatric neurosurgeon who is familiar with the medical aspects of myelomeningocele including its potentially positive aspects. For example, few children are profoundly retarded and most can compete in school. This discussion should be objective but not brutal. The initial counseling after the *in utero* diagnosis of spina bifida is usually done by the perinatologist who has never cared for a child or adolescent with spina bifida and who sees only the tragedy and loss and not the laughter and love. This is not, however, to underestimate the potential hardships that await the family. It is often helpful for the parents to meet other parents of children with spina bifida, or a child with the condition.

If possible, the mother should deliver at the tertiary care hospital where the child can receive definitive care. This maximizes the mother's ability to communicate with the baby's physicians, to bond with the baby, and to breast feed, if desirable.

Although still somewhat controversial, the preponderance of medical literature supports the routine delivery of babies with spina bifida by caesarean section.[5] Neurologic outcome appears better for children delivered by c-section than vaginally. This result is logical because the incidence of breech presentaion increases with spina bifida. Vaginal deliveries also increase the chance of applying traction on the neural placode, which is the termination of the spinal cord.

When the infant is not diagnosed *in utero* but is discoverd to have spina bifida at the time of routine delivery, whether vaginally or by c-section, the child will frequently have to be transferred to a tertiary center as soon as reasonable after birth, commonly within a few hours. During that period, the sac should be covered with a clean dressing and the baby kept prone in a heated incubator so the sac will not be traumatized. If this process is a lengthy one, intravenous broad spectrum antibiotics should be instituted.

If the mother and baby are stable, the mother should hold the baby for a short time before the transfer. The father should accompany the baby during the transport. The usual prenatal and natal information should accompany the baby as in the transport of any infant.

II. INITIAL EVALUATION OF THE NEWBORN

At the tertiary institution, the infant should be evaluated by an experienced neurosurgeon and pediatrician, either separately or together. The neurosurgeon will obviously be involved with the early repair of the sac, and if necessary, treatment of hydrocephalus. The pediatrician will be involved with the other aspects of the child at this time.

The pediatrician should take a careful history from one or both parents. This initial history can be therapeutic because the parents typically blame themselves for the deformity. The parents may be worrying about behaviors that might have caused the deformity, such as substance abuse or other activities contraindicated during pregnancy. These concerns should be elicited and addressed thoughtfully. The pediatrician can explain that the deformity occurred early in the pregnancy, at about 28 d of age, and that subsequent events had no effect.

A careful, general pediatric examination is necessary to assess the infant in general, as well as the specific lesions relating to myelodysplasia. Determining the presence of hydrocephalus, as indicated by an increased head circumference and large fontanel, is a key part of the initial examination. The sac should be examined to determine if it is intact or has ruptured during delivery. Its appearance, size, and position should also be observed. Deformities of the legs are the next priority. The presence of clubbed feet and the size of the legs should be noted. The legs must also be observed for movement because that information can help establish a preliminary prognosis about ambulation. If a sensory examination is performed to determine the level of neurological involvement, a spinal reflex to a pin prick, which often occurs with high level lesions, must be distinguished from a true response to pain. A sensory level with an infant responding to pain helps determine the level of the lesion and the prognosis for motor ability. The genitalia should be observed for urinary dribbling to determine continence. The appearance of the anus is also important in assessing fecal continence. Most children with myelodysplasia have a patulous anus with poor muscle tone that indicates involvment at the sacral level (S2-4) and problems with fecal continence.

After this initial assessment, the pediatrician should have an extensive discussion with both parents, if available. The mother, however, is commonly not present. If grandparents are present, they should be included in the discussion. The pediatrician should telephone the mother at the primary hospital. The call will establish a relationship, albeit long distance, on which to build long-term therapeutic communication. The call also relieves the father or another relative from the burden of relaying complicated and frightening information to a grieving mother.

Parents will have five basic questions about the infant that must be answered fully and honestly. Remember, however, that the amount of information that must be transmitted is overwhelming. It is not essential that all of this information be absorbed during the first interview.

1. What is the diagnosis, and what are the problems?
2. What caused the problem, and why did it happen to me?
3. What is the prognosis for function and life?
4. What should be done now and in the future?
5. Can it happen again in a subsequent pregnancy?

Usually, the pediatrician's role is to present the global picture of the infant, including the diagnosis and a brief explanation of the embryological mishap. It is important to stress that the cause of myelodysplasia is still unknown, despite numerous theories, and that it occurs very early in pregnancy. The procedures most apt to be done in the first hours of life should also be explained. For example, the major initial intervention, the closure of the sac, will usually occur within 24 h of birth. If hydrocephalus is apparent, many neurosurgeons will also insert a ventriculoperitoneal shunt or external ventriculostomy when the sac is repaired.

Parents will be anxious to know about the prognosis for ambulation. A reasonable assessment can usually be made from the initial examination. The inability of the child to maintain normal bowel and bladder control must be broached at this time and should include a brief statement that social continence can generally be attained using intermittent catheterization and a bowel-training regimen.

As more studies become available, the intellectual outlook for children with spina bifida becomes more positive.[6,7] Most children will have normal intelligence; with some assistance with their motor disabilities, most will attend normal classes in normal schools.

A discussion of the child's potential for sexual function is complicated and should initially be avoided. These issues are discussed in Chapter 8. If questions are asked, however, they should be answered honestly and openly. Unlike the potential for ambulation, the potential for sexual function, particularly among boys, is difficult to predict based on the initial examination. A growing number of young women with spina bifida have become mothers, and some young men with spina bifida have fathered children.[8]

Because many organ systems may be severely affected, parents will be overwhelmed initially. It is important to give parents a global picture with the best possible *realistic* prognosis. Describing the problem, but also offering remedies that will help the child become as normal as possible, provides realistic optimism and helps the parents to accept the child's condition. Special mention should be made of what is "right" about the baby, such as a healthy heart, strong lungs, or a good and vigorous appetite.

At this initial discussion, both parents should receive a similar prognosis and plan of early management. Therefore, it is essential that the neurosurgeon and pediatrician confer before discussing these aspects with the parents.

Commonly, the mother is unavailable for this initial discussion, which should therefore be repeated with her when she is able to visit the infant. Talking to both parents at the same time will help them have a common understanding. If grandparents or other relatives are going to be closely involved with the infant during early life, it is also helpful to include them in a similar discussion. Parents should be reassured that their questions are not foolish, that they are not expected to remember or understand all that is said, and that the information can be repeated at a later time as often as needed.

Frequently, siblings of the affected infant are forgotten during this period. They, too, would have been expecting a normal baby to arrive home with mother and will have many fears and misconceptions. Sometimes the pediatrician can help by discussing the baby with siblings if the parents are unable to do so adequately. Siblings should also visit the baby in the hospital a few days after the initial repair and be encouraged to bring a gift or something special to leave with the baby. The pediatrician should be alert to feelings of guilt if the sibling felt jealous or resentful during the pregnancy. All families have different strengths and handle events at different rates. Families who have children with spina bifida will also want to be congratulated on their new baby.

Parents are overwhelmed with the amount of information that must be absorbed. If too many people are involved during the first few days, they can become totally confused. We therefore recommend that other surgical specialties such as urologists and orthopedists do not discuss the infant with the parents during this early period. If surgical procedures, such as casting the clubfeet or treating dislocated hips are indicated during the initial hospital stay, the orthopedist should see the parents before treatment and discharge.

The pediatrician must understand the parental reaction to having a baby with significant deformities. Parents commonly go through several stages as described by Drotar et al. in their reaction to the news of a serious congenital malformation.[9] The initial parental reaction, disbelief and denial, is usually brief. The initial shock is also sometimes accompanied by anger projected at the physicians and a great deal of anxiety about their own ability to care for a deformed child. After a few days, a protracted period of sadness will last for weeks or months. After this prolonged period of depression, most parents will gradually adapt to their child's handicap and deal with it constructively. Drotar then describes a stage of reorganization characterized by gradual, positive, long-term acceapatance of the child. Achieving this stage is helped by parents' mutual support of each other. Throughout this process the pediatrician should demonstrate an understanding of the feelings expressed by the parents. The pediatrician will become an important person to the parents, so this acceptance and interest will help reestablish their self-esteem.

If an experienced, sensitive social worker is available, he or she can provide invaluable support to the parents. The social worker can frequently become involved during the first day or two of life and provide ongoing support that supplements the care given by nurses and physicians. Some parents are concerned about financial aspects of care, and the social worker can help obtain information on community or governmental resources. A social worker should also be expected to assist during family conflicts, when social supports are inadequate or absent, and when one or both parents have a history of emotional problems or cognitive deficits.

It is often helpful for the parents of a new baby with spina bifida to have the opportunity to talk to another parent who has already had the experience. This approach, however, must be individualized because some parents feel they must deal with the problems themselves. Most, however, are anxious to talk with someone. Parents need to understand that their baby has a future with special needs and problems and is not just a diagnosis. Talking to a family with a child with spina bifida will often help the parents acquire this perspective.

During this initial hospital stay, which generally lasts for 1 to 2 weeks, the neurosurgeon and pediatrician must communicate with the parents frequently. If a nurse coordinator will later be involved in the care of the child, he or she can facilitate this communication. Many booklets and pamphlets are available for parents of children with myelodvsplasia, but reading material should be screened carefully so parents do not receive too detailed an alarming picture during the first few days. These materials are available through the local chapter of the Spina Bifida Association of America (SBAA).

Urinary retention is a common problem in the immediate postoperative period. Frequently, a *Credé* maneuver (gentle pressure on the bladder transabdominally) performed every 3 to 4 h will alleviate the condition. If this procedure is needed for more than a few days, dilation of the ureters (hydroureter) may develop, and an indwelling Foley catheter will be required for a brief period.

The mother of a newborn with spina bifida should decide to breast feed independent of the birth defect. During the first 24 h while the surgical procedure and assessment are being performed, a breast pump may be necessary to start the flow of milk. Shortly after the repair, the child may be held on a pillow for breast feeding. In any case, the mother and father should be encouraged to hold the child as much as reasonable and to begin the process of caring for the baby while in the hospital.

Before discharge from the hospital, the hospital pediatrician should communicate so that a combined plan of management is understood by all concerned.

During the initial hospitalization a renal ultrasound is done to look for early hydronephrosis. In our experience, hydronephrosis is uncommon in the newborn but may develop during the first year of life or beyond. If significant hydronephrosis is present in this initial period, a urological consult is indicated.[10]

III. THE INFANT WITH SPINA BIFIDA AS AN OUTPATIENT

By 2 to 3 months of age, the infant should be examined by a multidisciplinary team consisting at minimum of a neurosurgeon, urologist, orthopedist, and pediatrician. Primarily, the pediatric role is to coordinate the care of the infant and to help the parents understand and utilize the information given by various surgical subspecialists. The plan of management must also be communicated to the family's local pediatrician so that he or she will be aware of the plans and treatments.

When the infant is 3 to 4 months of age, referral to a center that stimulates the infant by occupational and physical therapists can be very helpful. Mothers will frequently form a close relationship with the therapists, and this can assist the transition from sadness to adaptation. Physical therapy for the extremities may be indicated as prescribed by the orthopedist. In some centerrs, a small group of infants receive therapy together, and mothers can form a close relationship with other mothers of affected infants. In this setting, the pediatrician will be confronted by many questions comparing one infant to another. It is important to stress to the parents the unique treatment and prognosis for their child.

Some pediatricians will refer parents for genetic counseling after the first few months from birth. This advice can be helpful if parents are planning another pregnancy or if they are unusually concerned about the cause and prevention of myelodysplasia. Several studies have documented the value of giving multivitamins including folic acid before conception and during the first trimester. These studies[11,12] document a dramatic decrease in the expected incidence of this malformation. All couples contemplating pregnancy should be offered referral to a genetics center for counseling and prenatal diagnosis.

Many parents join a formal organization such as the local chapter of the SBAA. These groups can help give parents emotional support and educate them about the disease process and various treatments. The pediatrician on a myelodysplasia team is commonly involved in planning the educational programs with such groups.

IV. ROLE OF THE PEDIATRICIAN ON THE SPINA BIFIDA PLANNING TEAM

The child born with myelomeningocele is faced not only with the normal maintenance of health, termed "well child care" and the whole host of usual childhood illnesses, but also with a series of concerns unique to the abnormality. Managing these unique conditions, including skin protection, bowel management, obesity management, and specific psychosocial needs, is the responsibility of the team pediatrician and, often, the nurse coordinators working with the team.

Unless the family has continued to ask questions, to discuss the situation at home, and to study the written material distributed by either the clinic or the SBAA, much of the information shared with the parents will be forgotten. Depending on their orientation, families remember a few powerful statements, either positive or negative. Each visit with the pediatrician is an opportunity to review the educational aspects of spina bifida briefly, relative to its genetic aspects and the prognosis as it relates to this particular child. With time, the parent's questions will become more sophisticated, and their concerns must be addressed with a mixture of compassion and objectivity.

Pediatricians and social workers need to be aware of the psychological impact of the affected infant on the family. Some mothers will devote all of their enrgies to the care of this infant and neglect other members of the family, including the husband. This response can cause parental strife and also affect siblings. The period of sadness varies with each individual, but can last for months.

Parents should be encouraged at an early follow-up visit to reflect on what has gone well and what has been a problem in terms of family adaptation. Conflicts that arise from different parental coping patterns (i.e., one verbalizes feelings, the other "just keeps busy"; one is stoic, the other is demonstrative) should be addressed. The impact on social contacts and supports should also be explored, and suggestions should be offered for reconnecting with friends, family, and neighbors who may be too uncomfortable to make the first gesture. It is also helpful to give the parents a chance to identify what they have done well.

Although each individual has a different way to adapt to a child with myelodysplasia, some generalities should be remembered. Periods of depression commonly occur at major milestones in the development of the child: around the age when a normal child would begin to walk and to start kindergarten, and during early adolescence when parents become more concerned about the child's ability to be self-sufficient in adult life. These stages require further explanation and assessment.

Education of the child with spina bifida must be individualized. The Education of the Handicapped Act (PL 94-142) mandated that a child born with a handicap has a right between the ages of 3 to 21 to special education services and needs to receive education in the least restricitve environment possible. An amendment to this act in 1986 (PL 99-457) funded some early intervention services for children with handicaps between birth and 2 years old.[13] Most children with spina bifida may be educated in normal school classrooms with some special assistance. For example, younger children will need help from the school nurse with intermittent catheterization. Children with higher level lesions in wheelchairs or extensive bracing will require special adaptations in the classroom and may occasionally require education in orthopedically handicapped programs. Because most children with spina bifida have normal intelligence, the goal should be school in a regular classroom to further their integration into society.

Although most children with spina bifida have normal intelligence, many have difficulty with arithmetic and science. It is advisable to have a neuropsychologist test the child at the age of 5 to 6 years so that special learning disabilities can be recognized and addressed. The educational goal should be to maximize the student's potential (educationally as well as socially) so interaction with normal children in a regular classroom is encouraged as much as possible.

V. SKIN CARE

Because most infants with myelodysplasia have incompetent urinary and anal sphincters, they have much more difficulty with diaper rash. The usual preventive treatment of keeping infants as clean and dry as possible is recommended but is often unsatisfactory. The usual causes of diaper rash include monilial infection as well as general excoriation.

Throughout life one of the major problems for the child, adolescent, or adult with spina bifida is the prevention of pressure sores. For most of these children, the actual weight-bearing surfaces of their bodies (i.e., soles of the feet, buttocks) are anesthetic. These areas have poor circulation due to vasoparalysis and wounds therefore heal poorly.[14] Not only pressure, but also unrecognized heat can lead to full thickness skin loss in the feet and buttocks. Dangers include hot sidewalks, vinyl seat covers, car seat-belt buckles, and scalding bath water.[15]

As the children become ambulatory, pressure points on the feet can lead to callouses and decubitus ulcers. Prevention of ulceration by proper orthopedic and orthotic management is recommended, although sometimes ulceration is inevitable. Pressure sores may also occur in older children with a gibbus or those who sit in a wheelchair much of the time. Mothers must be instructed to observe these areas at least twice daily and to have the child lie prone until the erythema, if present, disappears. Teaching children to change their sitting position frequently is desirable but difficult to implement in the effort to prevent decubiti. Special cushions and adapted wheelchair seating are available and may be of great help.

During the school years, the child should begin to assume responsibility for his or her skin examination. Before entering the bathtub, the temperature of the water should be tested with the hand. After the bath, and every evening at least, the areas of potential pressure such as feet and buttocks should be thoroughly checked with mirrors.

When decubiti do appear, initial treatment is to keep pressure off the area and to keep it clean and dry. With only second-degree involvement, this management will suffice. However, when there is a sizable lesion of full skin thickness involvement, the lesions heal very, very slowly and commonly need a plastic surgical procedure such as a skin flap. Management of these lesions in the hospital for several days preoperatively includes cleansing procedures such as wet-to-dry dressings, which will also stimulate the vascular bed of the decubitus ulcer. Full-thickness lesions heal by regeneration of skin at the circumference of the lesion: consequently, the healing process is so slow that skin flaps are indicated. Simple skin grafts without subcutaneous tissue are usually short-lived because they break down quickly when pressure is applied. Complications of decubitus ulcers include osteomyelitis of the underlying bone, which is difficult to manage successfully.

VI. OBESITY

Obesity is one of the most difficult issues facing the patient with spina bifida. Except for children with purely sacral-level lesions with no motor disturbances whose only abnormalities involve bowel and bladder function, children with spina bifida must expend a greater degree of energy in ambulation than normal children. They are therefore less likely than normal children to participate in strenuous play and often tend toward sedentary lives. For children with some ankle function who ambulate with ankle-foot orthoses (AFOs) but who do not need crutches, sensible diet and encouraging major motor activities should be enough to maintain normal weight.

Normal people expend most calories by using large muscle groups of the lower extremities. When these muscles are paralyzed, as in children with thoracic and thoracolumbar-lesion levels, daily energy expenditures may be very low. These children tend to gain weight despite restrictive diets because they are unable to burn adequate calories using only the upper extremities.

As the child grows, the upper extremities strength requirements increase for the purposes of transfer and ambulation using crutches or canes. Obesity in this context will lead to a wheelchair existence earlier than if obesity had not occurred. The obese patient in a wheelchair is much less likely to live independently than the nonobese person in a wheelchair.

Extreme attention to the amount and quality of food ingested is essential to prevent obesity in these children. All caretakers should positively reinforce attempts by the child to limit the intake of sweets and fats. Interesting and enjoyable exercise programs tailored to the child's abilities should be developed and performed frequently. More research from exercise physiologists will be needed to find ways of attaining aerobic conditioning primarily using the upper extremities.

In patients with thoracic and thoracolumbar level lesions, scoliosis is quite common and makes determinations of height less useful. Weight-to-arm span recordings may be more realistic measures of obesity than weight-to-height measurements and may revel that the child is doing better than first assumed.

VII. BOWEL CARE

Almost all children with spina bifida lack sphincteric control of bowel function. In infancy, the biggest problem is constant soiling with loose stools leading to severe diaper rash. When the child is old enough to tolerate refined cereals and a low-fat diet, the change in diet will give the stool a firmer consistency and reduce the problem of diaper rash.

Usually the development of a bowel-training program, which will lead to fecal continence in most children with spina bifida, is delayed until the child is ready for preschool. Fecal continence is essential to the child's, and particularly to the adolescent's, self-esteem and ability to socialize adequately.[8,16] Failure to attain reasonable fecal continence leads to social isolation and ridicule.

A study done at Case Western Reserve University involving 94 patients with spina bifida over the age of 5 years revealed that two thirds (66%) were continent with only very occasional accidents. Another 19% had good control with less than one episode of soiling per week. This latter group was primarily composed of younger children. A small percentage (6%) were incontinent.[10]

For nonhandicapped children, the efforts toward fecal continence should begin between 18 to 30 months of age and are decidedly behavioristic. The toddler who can feel the urge to defecate is rewarded for performing this act in the toilet or potty chair with reasurring expressions. With time, the child is chastised for defecating in diapers or underwear. This combination of behavioral modification and neurologic maturation quickly leads to continence. For the child who does not sense the presence of stool in the colon, however, these

COMPARISON OF TWO MODELS OF BOWEL MANAGEMENT		
	Child Training	Colon Training
Goal	To use the toilet in response to the urge to defecate	To evacuate the colon of soft-formed stool at a predictable time
Baseline information	Neurological development Psychosocial development	Transit time Stool consistency Time of defecation
Onset	Toddlerhood	Infancy
Sensory cues	Abdominal discomfort	Not established
Enabling activities	Toilet the child Role model the behavior Encourage imitation Reward success	Manage diet, fluid intake, exercise, timing Optimum posturing Rectal stimulation
Self-care	Premised on comfort and pleasing	Premised on cognition

FIGURE 2. Comparison of two models of bowel management. (From Roberts, C. S., *BNI Q.*, 4(4): 37, 1988. With permission.)

techniques are futile. The emphasis on fecal continence must change from child- to colon-training (Figure 2).[16] Colon-training requires a thorough understanding of the physiology of colonic emptying and gastrointestinal reflexes. The cognitive nature of the process usually requires delaying the beginning of bowel-training until the child is ready to begin preschool (around 3 years of age).

More than any other therapeutic endeavor in the child with spina bifida, the development of a bowel program must be individualized. A multitude of potential mechanisms can be used to improve the possibility of fecal continence. Each will work for some but not all of these children. The most successful programs revolve around reserving time each morning or every other day to empty the colon completely. This effort may take between 15 and 60 min and should be undertaken 15 to 20 min after breakfast to utilize the gastrocolic reflex. The child then sits on the toilet and uses a variety of techniques to empty the lower colon, including blowing up balloons to increase intra-abdominal pressure, digital stimulation and extraction, enemas, or suppositories.[8,16]

Diet is extremely important in achieving fecal continence. High-fat diets, as found in most of the fast-food diets of adolescents, lead to rapid transit time with soft, unformed stools that make continence difficult if not impossible. Diet with a high bran and insoluble fiber content (fresh fruits and vegetables) will lend formed bulk to the stool and aid in the search for continence. For some children the use of specially formulated tape across the buttocks will help prevent constant soiling and odor. If one approach is too unpleasant or has failed, another should be tried.

VIII. ROLE OF THE COMMUNITY PEDIATRICIANS OR FAMILY PRACTITIONER

The presence of one or two children with spina bifida in a busy office practice can be a challenge for a pediatrician or family practitioner. It is essential that the role of the physician, as the child's doctor, be protected and encouraged. He or she will be asked to provide well child care and to deal with most of the child's normal childhood illnesses. The more information the team transmits to the practitioner, the more able he or she can deal with the issues confronting the developing handicapped child.

One issue of well child care relative to the spina bifida is the routine immunization with pertussis vaccine. Spina bifida and the Arnold-Chiari malformation complex represent a birth defect that occured at a single point in gestational development. The dynamic nature of these conditions relate to their effect on the growing child. As many as 15% of these children have a seizure disorder. All of this is static in the sense of the damage to the CNS. Opinion is reasonably uniform among caretakers that children born with spina bifida should receive DPT inoculations as recommended by the American Academy of Pediatrics for normal children.

Children with spina bifida are not exempt from normal diseases of childhood. The problem comes in distinguishing diseases of normal children from problems unique to this population.

Any child with spina bifida who develops a febrile illness should have a urinalysis and culture as a routine part of the work-up because urinary tract infections are an integral part of the condition. One of the biggest difficulties for the pediatricians in the community is distinguishing shunt-related problems from the usual diseases of childhood. Although no rule is absolute, some guidelines are helpful. Shunt infection is usually an operative complication. Most shunt infections occur within 2 months of surgery. Children who present with an unexplained febrile illness within the first 2 months of a shunt procedure should be presumed to have a shunt infection until one is excluded. The corollary is also important and somewhat reassuring. If a child has not had a shunt revision or shunt tap for a long time and presents with an illness that includes a significant fever, it is extremely unlikely to be shunt-related.

Viral gastroenteritis, which presents with irritability and vomiting, may mimic a shunt malfunction. In these situations it may be necessary to perform an imaging study (CT or MRI) and to have the child evaluated by a neurosurgeon. If fever and diarrhea are present, the diagnosis of shunt malformation is less likely and warrants a longer period of observation.

As health care becomes more expensive as it relates to the Gross National Product (GNP), and especially as it is reflected in the costs to employers providing insurance benefits to their employees, more emphasis is being placed on the rationing of health care services. In this context, the community pediatrician increasingly assumes the role of "gatekeeper" or "shepherd" of community resources. Spina bifida is extremely expensive, from the perspective of both health-care dollars expended and the out-of-pocket expenses of families.

If the pediatrician does assume the role of resourse-allocation supervisor, the relationship of the pediatrician to the team becomes extremely critical, and open lines of communication even more essential. The team must continuously make the pediatrician aware of its concerns about the child from a holistic approach. The therapeutic goals of the team must be agreed upon by all members of the team, which in an extended fashion include the child, the family, and the community pediatrician. Once the goals are established, the importance of expensive diagnostic tests and therapies to attaining the goals must be fully explained to the family and the community pediatrician. These therapies can include surgical procedures such as ankle fusions, or detethering procedures, or various orthotic devices.

Once the pediatrician understands the importance of the tests and therapies, he or she has the responsibility to act as the child's advocate to obtain these services. As emphasized throughout this book, an aggressive proactive posture relative to the treatment of children with spina bifida will lead to a higher likelihood that the child will reach the goals we all have for ourselves and each other, including a successful independent existence.

IX. ADOLESCENCE AND ADULTHOOD

The goal in the care of children with spina bifida is to maximize their potential to become well-adjusted, self-sufficient members of society. The lower the lesion level, the more likely this goal will be met; conversely, thoracic level lesions are very disabling and only the most determined individuals will become self-supporting adults. The pediatrician will continue to be important to the family, assisting them with long-range plans of care when the parents are aging.

Recreation is a major problem for adolescents and adults with thoracic or lumbar level lesions. The ability to drive an automobile opens many opportunities, and all but the most severely disabled should be evaluated for driving with special hand controls.

Education through high school is fairly straightforward. Some will select a work-study curriculum to prepare for entry directly into the work force in jobs that require minimal mobility (e.g., typist, file clerk, receptionist, telephone dispatcher). College preparation curricula are also realistic for many. Pediatricians who have worked with spina bifida children for years are constantly amazed at how independent many have become when they return home from college. A good vocational counselor is invaluable as a referral source at this stage of career development.

As with all adolescents, sexuality is of major importance. Commonly, the more disabled children will have been sheltered from the normal maturation process. The pediatrician should discuss sexuality with the parents and children throughout the school years as they do with normal children, realizing the limitations of the neurological lesion. Sexuality has its emotional components as well as the physical ones. Caring for another is healthy. Dating is just as important for people with spina bifida as it is for the able-bodied. Most girls and up to 25% of boys are fertile, but many factors must be weighed before parenthood is considered.

During infancy and early childhood, the pediatrician and team nurse (a person who is essential to a myelodysplasia team and who will assist the pediatrician with many of the tasks described throughout this chapter) will coordinate much of the care of the child by multiple specialists. The parents, however, are the most important members of the team, and they will gradually shoulder more of the responsibilites for communication and decision making as they become more knowledgeable. The pediatrician should cultivate this role of the parents during preschool and school years. As adolescence approaches, the young man or woman with spina bifida should assume more control of self-care as well as care given by professionals. Independence cannot be acquired suddenly. It is the result of a long continuum from early childhood.

If the ingredients of care have been successful through the years, the pediatrician now has assumed a new role, that of a respected counselor and friend.

REFERENCES

1. **Stein, S. C., Feldman, J. G., Friedlander, M., and Klein, R. J.,** Is myelomeningocele a disappearing disease?, *Pediatrics*, 69, 511, 1982.
2. **Adams, M. M., Greenberg, F., Khoury, M. J., Marks, J. S., and Oakley, G. P., Jr.,** Trends in clinical characteristics of infants with spina bifida, Atlanta, 1972-1979, *Am. J. Dis. Child*, 139, 514, 1985.
3. **Windham, G. C. and Edmonds, L. D.,** Current trends in the incidence of neural tube defects, *Pediatrics*, 70, 333, 1982.
4. **Khoury, M. J., Erickson, J. D., and James, L. M.,** Etiologic heterogeneity of neural tube defects: clues from epidemiology, *Am. J. Epidemiol.*, 115, 538, 1982.
5. **Garbaciak, J. A., Jr.,** Obstetrical issues in spina bifida: perinatal management, prevention, and surgery, *BNI Q.*, 4(4), 9, 1988.
6. **Mapstone, T. B., Rekate, H. L., Nulsen, F. E., Dixon, M. S., Jr., Glaser, N., and Jaffe, M.,** Relationship of CSF shunting and IQ in children with myelomeningocele: a retrospective analysis, *Child's Brain*, 11, 112, 1984.
7. **McLone, D. G., Czyzewski, D., Raimondi, A. J., and Sommers, R. C.,** Central nervous system infections as a limiting factor in the intelligence of children with myelomeningocele, *Pediatrics*, 70, 338, 1982.

8. **Liptak, G.S., Bloss, J. W., Briskin, H., Campbell, J. E., Hebert, E. B., and Revell, G. M.,** The management of children with spinal dysraphism, *J. Child Neurol.,* 3, 3, 1988.

9. **Drotar, D., Baskiewicz, A., Irvin, N., Kennell, J., and Klaus, M.,** The adaptation of parents to the birth of an infant with a congenital malformation: a hypothetical model, *Pediatrics,* 56, 710, 1975.

10. **Caldamone, A. A. and Dixon, M. S., Jr.,** *Current Trends in Urology,* Vol. 3, Williams & Wilkins, Baltimore, 93, 1985.

11. **Smithells, R. W., Seller, M. J., Harris, R., Fielding, D. W., Schorah, C. J., Nevin, N. C., Sheppard, S., Read, A. P., Walker, S., and Wild, J.,** Further experience of vitamin supplementation for prevention of neural tube defect recurrence, *Lancet,* 1, 1027, 1983.

12. **Milunsky, A., Jick, H., Jick, S. S., Bruell, C. L., MacLaughlin, D. S., Rothman, K. J., and Willett, W.,** Multivitamin/folic acid supplementation in early pregnancy reduces the prevalence of neural tube defects, *JAMA,* 262, 2847, 1989.

13. **Loda, C. G. and McCue G. E.,** Entitlement and discretionary programs for the disabled, *BNI Q.,* 4(4), 53, 1988.

14. **Hayden, P. W.,** Adolescents with myelomeningocele, *Pediatr. Rev.,* 6, 245, 1985.

15. **Gregg, S. A.,** Pediatric management of spina bifida: skin care, obesity, and psychosocial problems, *BNI Q.,* 4(4), 43, 1988.

16. **Roberts, C. S.,** Bowel management in spina bifida: perspectives and issues, *BNI Q.,* 4(4), 37, 1988.

Chapter 4

THE CHIARI MALFORMATION ASSOCIATED WITH MYELOMENINGOCELE

May L. Griebel, W. Jerry Oakes, and Gordon Worley

TABLE OF CONTENTS

I. INTRODUCTION

The hindbrain hernia described as the Chiari malformation and occurring with myelomeningoceles has a spectrum of pathological changes, but frequently has the following principal anatomic features:

1. Caudal displacement of the cerebellar vermis through the foramen magnum
2. Caudal displacement and elongation of the medulla oblongata and sometimes the pons
3. Caudal displacement of the cervical spinal cord
4. Kinking of the medulla
5. Obliteration of the cisterna magnum[42,47]

With advances in the treatment of the complications associated with spina bifida, particularly renal disease,[22] problems resulting from brain stem dysfunction associated with the Chiari malformation have arisen as a leading cause of mortality and serious, newly acquired, secondary morbidity in children with myelomeningocele.[25,26,29] In our experience[34] and that of others,[18] the clinical presentation of Chiari-related problems depends upon the age of the child. Infants present predominantly with signs and symptoms of medullary dysfunction while older children and adolescents present with evidence of cervical cord disease and cerebellar dysfunction. Approximately one third of children born with a myelomeningocele develop potentially life-threatening symptoms of brain stem dysfunction. For most, the symptoms resolve, but a third of those with symptoms die (12% of the total).

Because of the variability of outcome, controversy surrounds the approaches to therapy. In this chapter on the Chiari malformation associated with myelomeningocele, we discuss the historical perspective, the pathological anatomy, embryogenesis, clinical presentation, evaluation, surgical technique for posterior fossa decompression and laminectomy, and outcome.

II. HISTORICAL PERSPECTIVE

The description of herniation of posterior fossa contents through the foramen magnum was probably first done by Cleland in 1883. This summary of the pathological findings of a single patient with a myelomeningocele did not devote itself to the hindbrain herniation and there lies the reason Cleland is usually given little credit in our understanding of this entity. Chiari in publications in the 1890s first called our attention to the specific entity and subsequently categorized four types or degrees of hindbrain herniation or deformity.

Type I: Caudal displacement of the cerebellar tonsils through the foramen magnum without significant herniation or deformity of the lower brain stem or fourth ventricle

Type II: Caudal displacement of the inferior portion of the cerebellar vermis, the medulla, and lower pons, and an elongated fourth ventricle through the foramen magnum

Type III: Caudal displacement of the inferior cerebellum and brain stem into a high cervico-occipital myelomeningocele

Type IV: Hypoplasia of the cerebellum without displacement of posterior fossa contents

Although intermediate or hybrid patients have been reported, Chiari's delineation remains useful both clinically and pathologically. The Type II lesion with displacement of cerebellar vermis, brain stem, and the fourth ventricle is usually associated with the myelomeningocele population.

Arnold's name was added to the eponym by Schwalbe and Gredig in 1907. Writing from Arnold's laboratory they utilized the term "Arnold-Chiari malformation" to describe patients with Type II deformity. This term became popular and is still used extensively today. The inclusion of Arnold's name seems somewhat unwarranted in light of his limited contribution.

III. PATHOLOGICAL ANATOMY

The Chiari II malformation is almost always associated with a myelomeningocele and involves a more complex and extensive set of anomalies of the hindbrain, cervical spinal cord, and craniovertebral junction than are seen with the Chiari I malformation. Basic to the disturbed anatomy is a variable caudal displacement of the inferior cerebellar vermis, lower brain stem, and fourth ventricle. The foramen magnum is abnormally enlarged whereas the posterior fossa is much smaller than usual and the floor of the posterior fossa may be unusually flat (platybasia). The tentorium cerebelli is hypoplastic and attaches quite caudally. The incisura is abnormally widened and elongated because of underdevelopment of the tentorial leaves. The transverse sinuses and torcula may be so displaced that they lie within 2 to 3 cm of the rim of the foramen magnum. The petrous ridges and clivus are commonly scalloped, again reflecting the crowding of the posterior fossa. Naidich, who has written extensively on the subject, believes that the petrous erosion increases directly with the cerebellar growth.[29-32]

The mesencephalon is virtually always abnormal (Figure 1), being beaked and elongated posteriorly. In the mildest form, the four colliculi are separate entities, but the quadrigeminal plate is shortened and the inferior two colliculi are elongated sagittally. At the other extreme, the colliculi are all fused into a conical mass with beaking of the tectum,[11] the apex of which rests between the cerebellar hemispheres. The pineal gland may be posteriorly elongated. The cerebellum, in addition to its caudal displacement, bulges rostrally through the incisura to sit above the hypoplastic tentorium. Upward displacement of the cerebellum is particularly marked after shunting of the lateral ventricles and has been demonstrated in more than half of patients after shunt placement. In

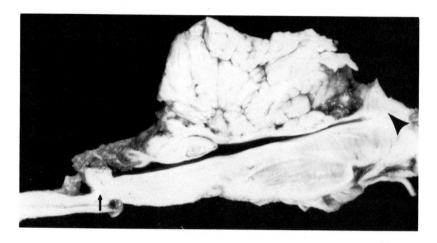

FIGURE 1. Gross pathology of beaked quadrigeminal plate. Midsagittal autopsy specimen of the brain stem, cerebellum, and upper cervical spinal cord of a child with a Chiari malformation associated with myelomeningocele. Caudal descent of the cerebellar vermis, fourth ventricle, and lower brain stem is apparent. The extraventricular position of the choroid plexus lying on the medullary kink (arrow) is also seen. Beaking of the quadrigeminal plate is seen immediately to the right of the cerebellum.

this position it may act as an extra-axial mass and displace other normal structures (Figure 2). Cerebrospinal fluid (CSF) pools around the towering cerebellum in what has been called the pericerebellar cistern.[31]

Another change in the supratentorial cerebellum is that its anterior margins tend to roll over, creating an undulating anterior cerebellar surface. Below the tentorium the cerebellum also becomes displaced and grows forward to creep around the lateral borders of the brain stem (an inverted cerebellum). Its margins may even meet in the anterior midline and cover the basilar artery. As the cerebellum grows lateral to the midbrain, it overlaps the cerebral peduncles and can eventually separate the midbrain from the hippocampus. As it grows lateral to the pons, the cerebellum bulges into the cerebellopontine angle cisterns and can present radiographically as bilateral cerebellopontine angle "masses". The portion of the cerebellum that herniates caudally varies from having no tissue below the foramen magnum in 10% of patients to having the great horizontal fissure extend below the foramen in 18%. The length of the cerebellar tail has no relationship to the length of the medullary hernia but does vary inversely with the age of the child and overall cerebellar weight. The strangulation effect invariably produces atrophy in the cerebellar tail, and the nodulus may be almost totally necrosed in severe cases.[32]

The Chiari II fourth ventricle is flattened and elongated with no apparent lateral recesses and it may extend into the cervical spinal canal. Venes et al.[49] described three types of fourth ventricular deformity based on preoperative magnetic resonance imaging (MRI) or intraoperative ultrasound studies (Figure 3). In Type A, the fourth ventricle is not dilated but continues caudally as

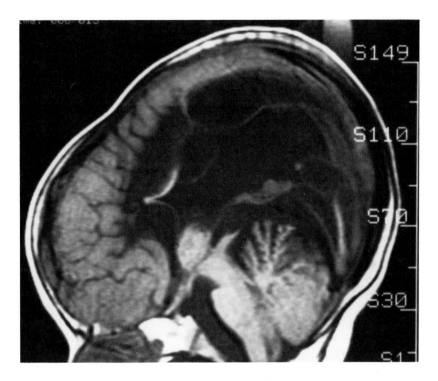

FIGURE 2. MRI of high riding cerebellum. Midsagittal MRI of an infant with a myelomeningo-cele and dysplastic medial occipital and parietal lobes. Abundant CSF space medial to both hemi-spheres lies immediately above the cerebellum.

a narrow canal below the foramen magnum. Type B consists of intracranial dilatation of the fourth ventricle and the aqueduct with variable intraspinal extension of the cystic fourth ventricle. In Type C, there is intraspinal dilatation of the fourth ventricle wihout intracranial dilatation, generally lying such that the long axis of the cyst is dorsal to but aligned with the spinal canal. The position of the choroid plexus varies and it may reside in its embryologic position outside the fourth ventricle.

Cystic dilatation of the fourth ventricle appears to be associated with de-formity of the medulla such that in ~70% of patients as the medulla descends, it buckles downward and backward to a variable degree to form a cervicome-dullary kink. The buckling usually occurs just inferior to the gracile and cuneate tubercles, so that they point caudally and form the apex of the spur. Portions of the upper cervical spinal cord typically descend with the medulla, and thus C1 and C2 may lie dorsal and caudal to C3 and C4. Emery and MacKenzie[13] defined five degrees of deformity ranging from a mild inferior displacement of the spinal cord to severe buckling of the medulla with a diverticulum of the fourth ventricle dorsally (Figure 4). Most commonly there is less than 5 mm of overlap of the medulla on the spinal cord. Although the

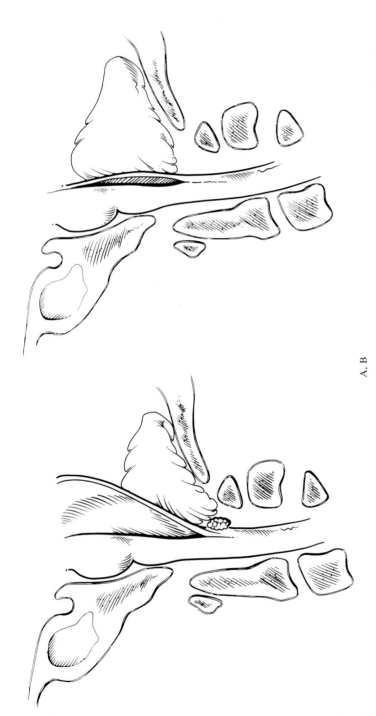

A, B

FIGURE 3.   Three types of the fourth ventricle after Venes. Artist's rendition of the various cranio-cervical anomalies described by Venes.[49] (A) Caudal descent of the cerebellar vermis with occlusion of the foramen of Magendie by fibrovascular adhesions. (B) Caudal descent of the cerebellar vermis associated with dilatation of the fourth ventricle. (C-1) Cystic enlargement of the caudal aspect of the fourth ventricle dorsal to the upper cervical spinal cord. (C-2) The entire cerebellum and fourth ventricle is seen to lie within the cervical spine. This may be associated with syringo-hydromyelia.

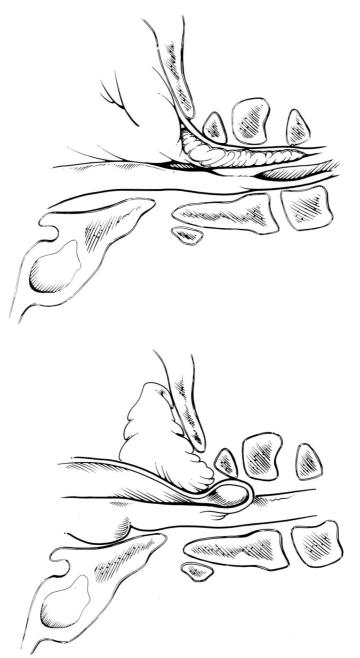

FIGURE 3C, D.

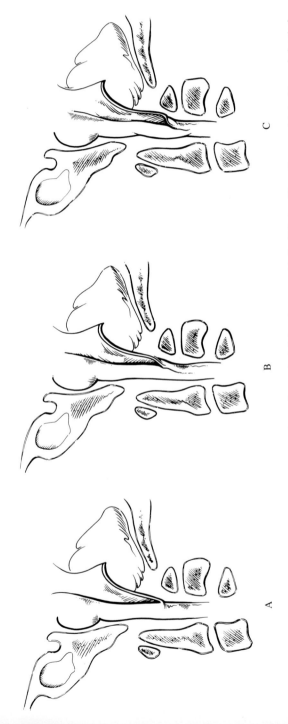

FIGURE 4.   Medullary kink degrees. Depiction of the degrees of medullo-cervical dislocation seen with the Chiari malformation associated with myelodysplasia. These range from mild descent of the fourth ventricle with minimal buckling of the medulla (A) to severe cystic expansion and displacement of the fourth ventricle associated with severe kinking and encystment of the most caudal portion of the displaced ventricle (E). (After Emory and McKenzie.[13])

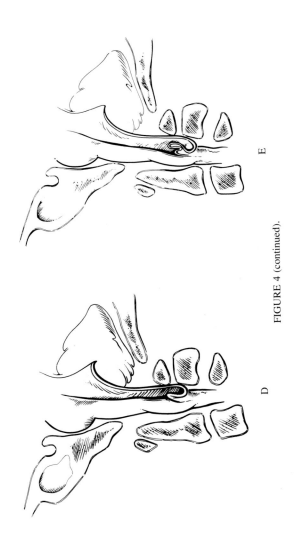

FIGURE 4 (continued).

spur usually lies between C2 and C4, it may be located as low as the upper thoracic level. With the descent of the medulla and even of the pons, the lower cranial nerves may be forced to ascend through the foramen magnum before exiting.

With the cascade of downward herniation of the cerebellum, fourth ventricle, and brain stem, cervical spinal cord segments, especially C3 to C6, become compressed, are shorter than usual, and are flattened sagitally and broadened transversely. The length of the dentate ligaments may help to determine the degree of medullary overlap and subsequent compression of the cord. Short and abnormally thickened dentate ligaments may anchor the cord high and allow only minimal caudal excursion. Attachment of the shortened first dentate ligaments to the foramen magnum in effect forms a sling behind which the medulla herniates. The central canal typically is abnormal and may be associated with hydromyelia in up to 95%[5] of cases or with a communicating syringomyelia.[32]

Associated with the cervicomedullary abnormalities of the Chiari II malformation are a number of supratentorial anomalies which were detailed by Peach.[42] These include hydrocephalus with enlargement of the lateral ventricles, especially of the atria and occipital horns. In contrast, the third ventricle commonly is mildly dilated. Also described are cerebral heterotopies with nodules projecting into the ventricles, thickening of the massa intermedia, fenestrations or absence of the septum pellucidum, craniolacunia or "lückenschädel" of the skull, hypoplasia or fenestration of the falx cerebri, polygyria, and histological derangement of the cerebral cortex into four rather than six layers. Although major cortical anomalies are common, the vast majority of patients have the potential for normal intellectual function.[24,25] Bony anomalies of the spinal column include diastematomyelia, hemivertebrae, and spina bifida, among others.

IV. EMBRYOGENESIS

Although both Chiari malformations I and II have been extensively studied, there is no uniform opinion regarding their embryogenesis. Theories that have been advanced to explain their occurrence generally have fallen into four categories:

1. Traction on the hindbrain by tethering of the spinal cord at the myelomeningocele causes the herniation
2. Expanding hydrocephalus "pushes" the hindbrain caudally
3. There is a local developmental anomaly with dysgenesis or arrest of development which causes expulsion of the hindbrain from the posterior fossa; included here are the possibilities of a differential growth rate between the bony and nervous structures and of an abnormally long hindbrain because of failure of formation of the pontine flexure

4.   The herniation is secondary to a tissue-pressure gradient between the intracranial contents and those of the spinal theca

The traction theory was proposed by Penfield and Coburn[43] in 1938 and strongly supported by Lichtenstein[23] in 1942. The flaws in this theory include the fact that angulation of the spinal roots is normal in the thoracic region and abnormal in the cervical region, which is difficult to explain based on lumbrosacral or lower thoracic tethering. The S-shaped deformity of the medulla and upper cervical cord implies an overgrowth or downward displacement of tissue, whereas with tethering one would expect attenuation of these tissues. Traction, likewise, cannot explain the upward herniation of the cerebellum, the beaking of the quadrigeminal plate, nor the supratentorial anomalies seen with the Chiari II malformation.

Chiari believed that hydrocephalus caused the hindbrain deformity of the Chiari II malformation, similar to the manner in which increased intracranial pressure causes cerebellar herniation in an adult. While this theory can explain the persistence of herniation in the face of hydrocephalus, it does not explain its development. Cases of congenital hydrocephalus without myelodysplasia do not display the hindbrain anomaly. Also, the Chiari II malformation is not invariably accompanied by hydrocephalus.

The idea that a local developmental anomaly causes expulsion of the hindbrain has been proposed by several authors. Patten[40] thought that localized overgrowth of the formative hindbrain was responsible for the deformity. A major flaw in this theory is that instead of being hyperplastic, as would be expected based on this explanation, the cerebellum in the Type II Chiari malformation is hypoplastic and poorly differentiated. Daniel and Strich[8] and later Peach[41] postulated that the Chiari II deformity was due to developmental arrest with failure of the pontine flexure to form during early embryonic life, leading to marked elongation of the brain stem. They then hypothesized that upward movement of the brain stem would cause changes such as beaking of the tectum. Caudal herniation of the medulla and vermis below the foramen magnum could likewise result from elongation of the brain stem. Peach felt that there was a critical time for fusion of the neural tube and that if fusion did not occur at this stage, further growth might be excessive. Thickening of the massa intermedia, polygyria, diastematomyelia, and craniolacunia fit into his theory as an arrest of development with subsequent faulty maturation and hypertrophy of the remaining elements. Again, this theory can be criticized because of the typically seen hypoplastic cerebellum. Also, while this is an attractive way to pull together the wide variety of anomalies that are seen in conjunction with the Chiari II malformation, it cannot explain the Chiari I anomaly nor the dynamics of the progressive development of symptoms in a Chiari II malformation.

Cameron[5] proposed the tissue-pressure gradient model, saying that the hindbrain hernia is caused by pressure disturbances rsulting from leakage of CSF from myelomeningocele into the amniotic cavity. The fluid leak would cause the cranium and its contents to be subjected to relatively increased amniotic pressure. Emery and MacKenzie[13] supported this concept when they found that the degree of deformity of the craniocervical junction was proportional to the extent of the myelomeningocele, saying that with a larger defect there would be a greater pressure gradient and thus increased hindbrain malformation. Welch et al.,[51] Williams,[52] and Newman et al.[33] applied Cameron's model of tissue-pressure gradient in explaing the development of the Chiari I malformation in patients both with and without spinal shunts. Welch described four patients who developed the Chiari I deformity years after lumboperitoneal shunt insertion and who did not have the hindbrain hernia by radiographic or direct visualization prior to their shunting. Consequently, he questioned whether the anomaly could be acquired. Welch noted the presence of spinal mechanisms for the absorption of CSF by spinal arachnoid villae associated with spinal nerve roots into dural venous sinusoids. If cephalic mechanism for absorption of CSF were impaired, either spinal shunting or maintenance of function in the spinal absorptive pathway could lead to occurrence of a Chiari I anomaly secondary to a pressure gradient between the cranial and spinal compartments. This gradient would not be large but would be exacerbated by the upright posture, requiring years for the development of a symptomatic deformity. Whether a similar mechanism exits *in utero* causing the more severe Chiari II deformity remains speculative.

The development of hindbrain hernias associated with myelodysplasia has been investigated by examining affected embyos and fetuses of various gestational ages. Osaka et al.[37] found that the intrauterine formation of the hindbrain anomaly followed the development of the myelomeningocele. Since development of the cerebellar vermis precedes development of the cerebellar hemispheres and tonsils, embryological intracranial and intraspinal pressure differences could result in caudal displacement of the vermis first.

Williams[52] lent further support to the differential pressure theory by simultaneously measuring CSF pressure within the cranial cavity and spinal canal, both in patients with symptomatic type I Chiari malformations and in normal controls. A Valsalva maneuver causes intraspinal pressure to increase because of engorgement of the epidural veins. Compression of the spinal subarachnoid space leads to cephalic movement of the pressure wave and CSF into the intracranial cavity. With relaxation there is outflow from the intracranial cavity and then the spinal venous pressure returns to normal. If the pressure equilibration is delayed by adhesions and/or tissue in the foramen magnum, a pressure differential between the intracranial and intraspinal fluid compartments is created. Alternative pathways of decompression are then encouraged, including reduction of pressure through a patent obex and progressive caudal herniation of the tissue at the foramen magnum. In patients with type I Chiari malformation, the relaxation phase of intracranial pressure is prolonged. In very symptomatic patients, a pressure gradient may even be documented at rest. This type study has not been performed in the typical myelomeningocele population with the Chiari II malformation. Like Williams, Gardner[15] focused on CSF hemodynamics as the mechanism for dysraphism, especially for the origin of syringomyelia associated with the Chiari malformations. The normal outlets of the fourth ventricle, the foramina of Luschka and Magendie, remain functionally closed because of delay in their embryological opening with late or inadequate rupture of the rhombic roof. The natural egress of CSF from the fourth ventricle is obstructed and the pulsatile flow of CSF creates a "water-hammer" pulse effect which can be dissipated through a patent obex into the the central canal of the spinal cord. Although it is not clear whether the intracranial-intraspinal pressure gradient is caused primarily by inadequate perforation of the embryonic rhombic roof or by a time-sensitive arrest of neural tube closure, a combination of the hemodynamic and pressure differential theories provides an attractive explanation for the formation of the Chiari malformations. This mechanism alone has significant difficulty in explaining every finding seen in association with Chiari II malformations. Some dysgenetic component must also be present in some patients.[17] However, dysgenetic features would not easily help us understand progressive symptoms that can clearly be present in this patient population.

V. CLINICAL PRESENTATION

In our experience[34,35] and in that of others,[2,18] the pattern of clinical presentation of Chiari-related problems depends upon the age of the child. Infants present predominantly (but not exclusively) with signs and symptoms of brain stem dysfunction, while older children and adolescents have cervical spinal cord or cerebellar dysfunction. The patterns are not mutually exclusive. Cervical spinal cord symptoms occur in some infants presenting with brain stem dysfunction and older children with cord symptoms may also have brain stem dysfunction.[47]

Infants may be born with medullary dysfunction, but more commonly develop it within the first 2 months of life.[2,45] The peak mortality from Chiari-related problems due to brain stem dysfunction is between 9 and 12 weeks of age.[50] Infants with a low level myelomeningocele and, therefore, a better prognosis for ambulation and independent life than others, are more frequently affected than those with extensive spinal cord lesions.[19,20] Life-threatening symptoms result from dysfunction of cranial nerves IX and X and the medullary respiratory center.[19,21,25,44,45,47,50] Mild inspiratory stridor when crying is usually the premonitory symptom. It results from paresis of the vocal cord abductors.[3,19] As stridor worsens, obstructive apnea may develop[50] due to vocal cord paralysis. Involvement of medullary respiratory center may result in apnea and bradycardia (in the absence of obstruction at the vocal cords), increased proportion of periodic breathing during sleep, and ventilatory insensitivity to marked hypercapnea, all of which have been documented in infants with myelomeningocele.[50] Absent sleep arousal to increased CO_2 concentration has also been reported.

Another life-threatening problem of infants with myelomeningocele is aspiration pneumonia caused by palatal and/or pharyngeal dysfunction, often associated with gastroesophageal reflux.[25,39] Esophageal dismotility has been reported in infants with myelomeningocele and other Chiari-related symptoms[16,25,39] and is probably related to vagal nerve dysfunction.

In addition to these problems, infants and older children may also have clinically evident involvement of other lower cranial nerves. Facial diplegia, weakness of the sternocleidomastoid, and tongue fasciculations have all been reported.[45,48]

Potentially lethal breath-holding spells may develop in infancy or early in childhood. These spells, in common with breath-holding spells in neurologically normal children, are often provoked by anger. The child then develops obstructive apnea, turns cyanotic, and loses consciousness. Spontaneous respirations resume spontaneously after loss of consciousness but convulsions or death may occur.

Tomita and McLone[47] reported three school-aged children who developed neck pain and occipital headache followed reportedly by respiratory arrest, presumably due to respiratory medullary center dysfunction. All children had hydrocephalus and shunt dysfunction. Prompt resolution of symptoms occurred with shunt revision.

Cervical spinal cord dysfunction is the most common mode of presentation of Chiari-related symptoms in older children and adolescents, although paresis and sensory abnormalities may also occur in infants. These abnormalities may be due to the Chiari malformation per se or may be the result of an associated syrinx.[4] Infants may have arm weakness and spasticity, as well as retrocollis and opisthotonus. Older children present with progressive upper extremity weakness and loss of fine motor control. Suspended and dissociated sensory loss may also occur. Upper extremity deep tendon reflexes become more brisk. With further progression, flexion contractures of the fingers with marked atrophy of all muscles of the upper extremity develop. The cervical spinal cord dysfunction associated with the Chiari malformation often present as an increased amount of time and effort needed to perform activities of daily living (such as tieing shoes), gradually progressing to incapacity.

Rarely, children with symptomatic Chiari malformations present principally with progressive truncal and appendicular ataxia. In our series,[35] only 2 of 29 patients who had posterior fossa decompression and laminectomy for Chiari-related symptoms had this pattern of clinical involvement as the reason for surgery.

As mentioned, Chiari-related symptoms may be provoked by increased intracranial pressure[47] but they also occur in its absence.[21,49] Different factors may be involved in the pathogenesis of symptoms in different patients. The brain stem itself may be dysmorphic, resulting in dysfunction and symptoms.[17] The disorganized brain stem may also be more sensitive to compression by hydrocephalus.[2,19] Medullary hemorrhages, recent and old, have been found at autopsy in children who died of respiratory problems.[28,42] In one series, 13 of 14 infants with myelomeningocele who died of respiratory symptoms had evidence of a medullary vascular lesion (hemorrhage, hemorrhagic necrosis, or bland infarct) compared to 0 of 15 who did not have respiratory problems but died from another cause.[38] The normal posterior fossa architecture is distorted by the Chiari malformation, perhaps predisposing to vascular lesions.[10,12] A paucity of neurons in the nucleus ambiguous with degeneration of those remaining has also been reported.[3,7] Traction on the cranial nerves as they ascend from their abnormal caudal position toward the intracranial foramen of exit has also been found at autopsy[42] and may be a factor causing dysfunction.[3]

Although almost all children with myelomeningocele have an associated Chiari II malformation,[8] only 20 to 40% will develop Chiari-related signs and symptoms.[25,39] About one third who develop symptoms will die. For the rest, symptoms resolve spontaneously over time or do not progress to death.

Because the natural history is variable, there is controversy about the approach to management of brain stem symptoms in infants and children. One general principle, however, is accepted: the first step is to be sure that intracranial pressure is not increased. If it is, the child needs a functional shunt. Shunt revision can result in prompt resolution of symptoms.[36,47] However, symptoms may persist in the presence of normal intracranial pressure. Infants with a functional shunt whose symptoms are not progressive or life-threatening can certainly be observed over time. Children with intermittent stridor or even stridor continuously present at rest in no distress can be observed. If stridor progresses to respiratory distress or if apnea and bradycardia develop, more aggressive management is indicated. In our series, each of the patients undergoing posterior fossa decompression and laminectomy for brain stem symptoms related to the Chiari malformation had one or more of the following indications for surgery:

1. Stridor continuously present at rest resulting in respiratory distress
2. Recurrent aspiration pneumonia (two or more episodes) caused by palatal dysfunction and/or gastroesophageal reflux
3. Life-threatening apnea and bradycardia
4. Cyanotic breath-holding spells resulting in loss of conciousness occasionally requiring resuscitation

If stridor and feeding difficulties persist after decompression, then gastrostomy, fundoplication, and occasionally tracheostomy may be indicated. A pneumogram obtained after posterior fossa decompression and laminectomy may be useful in determining if the apnea has resolved. If it has not, home apnea monitoring of children and cardiorespiratory resuscitation training for parents should be considered.

In contrast to the controversy surrounding the management of brain stem

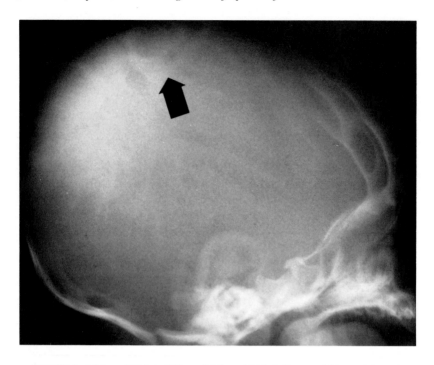

FIGURE 5. Lückenschädel skull X-ray. Lückenschädel skull or cranial lacunae (arrow).

symptoms related to the Chiari malformation, there is agreement that the symptoms attributed to cervical spinal cord dysfunction are relieved by posterior fossa decompression and laminectomy.[35,36] Some children with severe truncal and/or appendicular ataxia may also improve after posterior fossa decompression and laminectomy.

VI. EVALUATION

Although techniques for assessment of a possible Chiari malformation have grown increasingly sensitive, the initial evaluation should still include routine roentgenograms of the skull and cervical spine. This should include dynamic flexion-extension views of the cervical spine to assess stability.

Skull films of the child with a Chiari malformation associated with myelomeningocele are likely to demonstrate Lückenschädel, or craniolacunae, in at least 85% of patients.[42] This is most marked in the upper half of the calvaria, immediately beneath the vertex. This finding may be seen until 6 months of age when it usually disappears completely whether or not there is progressive hydrocephalus.[29] Lückenschädel (Figure 5) appears as thinnings or pits in the membranous bone affecting both the inner and the outer aspects of the calvaria. According to Naidich, mild Lückenschädel is seen more readily on CT than on skull films. Brain tissue can be demonstrated to bulge into the pits. Other findings include erosion of the petrous pyramids, enlargement of the foramen magnum, elongation of the laminar arches of the upper cervical vertebrae, small size of the posterior fossa with caudal attachment of the tentorium, basilar impression, platybasia, Klippel-Feil deformity, and hemivertebrae.

Evaluation of hindbrain and cervicomedullary pathology is being revolutionized by the application of MRI, which is currently the optimum methodology of delineating the anatomy (Figure 6B). In the past, techniques to obtain contrast studies have included ventriculography, pneumencephalography, and positive contrast or air myelography. Angiography has been utilized to demonstrate the descent of the tonsillar loop of the posterior inferior cerebellar artery. CT scanning of the head to assess ventricular size and position is important since hydrocephalus can be seen in greater than 85% of myelomeningocele patients and can be followed readily by CT. Water soluble cisternography has recently been utilized as a powerful diagnostic tool[14] (Figure 6A). Delayed migration of contrast within the substance of the spinal cord facilitates the diagnosis of syringomyelia, and the contrast is also quite precise in allowing definition of the structures in the cervical canal. Drawbacks to this type of evaluation include the need for lumbar puncture with injection of a potentially toxic substance intrathecally, the requirement for hospitalization of some patients, technical problems of bony artifact in the posterior fossa and spinal canal, and poor spatial resolution of reformatted images. MRI has repeatedly been shown to demonstrate clearly the pathology of the Chiari malformations, including intramedullary cystic dilatations.[1,9,27] This obviates the need for cisternography in many patients. MRI can provide better tissue contrast than water soluble cisternography and is not subject to bony artifact.

The question remains of how to evaluate the contribution of a documented Chiari malformation to the symptomatology with which a patient presents. The role of brain stem and somatosensory evoked potentials (SSEPs), electronystagmography, prolonged esophageal pH probes (Tuttle test), barium swallow, and CO_2 response curves is now being evaluated.[26,35] Normalization of brain stem auditory evoked potentials has correlated with clinical improvement in a limited number of patients following posterior fossa decompression for symptomatic Chiari malformations.[26,46] Likewise, SSEPs have been shown to normalize following decompression.[16] This suggests that evoked potentials may provide useful objective parameters in some patients by which to measure progression of symptoms and surgical benefit. Similar findings have occurred with CO_2 curves.[35] Oakes et al.[35] documented a significant improvement on hypercapnic ventrilatory drive in seven of ten patients who had a CO_2 response test performed before and after posterior fossa decompression and laminectomy.

VII. SURGICAL MANAGEMENT

Given that hydrocephalus and clinical evidence of increased intracranial

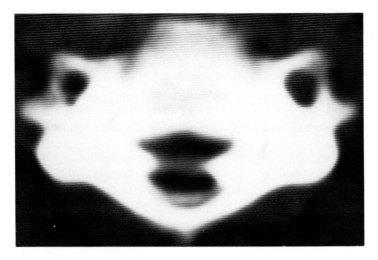

A

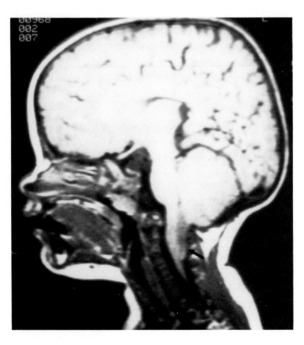

B

FIGURE 6. Cisternogram CT and MRI (Chiari I, II). (A) CT myelogram of the upper cervical spine showing two (dark) elliptical filling defects in the (white) subarachnoid space. The upper, more flattened ellipse is the cervical spinal cord while the more rounded dorsal defect represents the displaced cerebellar vermis. (B) Midsagittal MRI of a child with a myelomeningocele. Descent of the darker cerebellar vermis (arrow) dorsal to the spinal cord is seen well below the plane of the foramen magnum. At operation the vermis was ischemic.

pressure are seen in a significant number of patients with symptomatic Chiari malformations, the initial procedure of choice is normalization of the intracranial pressure by means of a valve-regulated ventricular shunt. This should be done as expeditiously as possible. Shunting alone may cause symptoms to recede.

Unfortunately, this is clearly a minority of symptomatic patients. In the situation of a functioning shunt and normal intracranial pressure, consideration should be given to direct decompression of the cranio-cervical junction.

Intraoperative positioning is critical, and care must be taken not to excessively flex the neck. Tetraplegia secondary to spinal cord compression has been seen as a consequence of excessive flexion, especially in patients with basilar impression.[49] The suboccipital craniectomy is much more limited than those performed for exploration of midline posterior fossa lesions. The thickened bone at the edge of the foramen magnum and the thickened atlanto-occipital membrane, which may be tenaciously attached to the edge of the foramen magnum, must be carefully removed. Opening the dura of the posterior fossa in neonates and young infants is considered only after the cervical dura is open. It is important to remember that the transverse sinus may actually be near the foramen magnum. The risk of the opening is contrasted with the potential benefit of the decompression as one proceeds cephalad. The vast majority of the compression occurs either at the foramen magnum or under the arch of C1. In our experience, there has not been the need to extend the bony or dural opening more than 1 to 2 cm cephalad of the foramen magnum.

The laminectomy performed must extend to below the level of the herniated cerebellar tissue. As noted by Venes et al.,[49] the pathology lies in the midline, and thus care should be taken to remove only those bony elements necessary for exposure of the displaced cerebellum and brain stem. Especially in the presence of syringomyelia, cervical laminectomy carries a significant risk of progressive kyphosis. It is not necessary to remove additional bone to expose the caudal extent of an associated syrinx.

The dura and arachnoid are commonly thickened with adhesions at the level of the maximum constriction. In addition, a tight fibrous extradural band may occur, usually at the level of C1, and its section can provide immediate relief of compression. Identation can actually be demonstrated on the underlying tissue (Figure 7). Dense subarachnoid adhesions are also commonly present, and their dissection carries with it significant risk for damage to vital vascular and neural structures. One must weigh the risk of dissection vs. the benefit of providing free egress of fluid from the fourth ventricle. Small branches of the posterior inferior cerebellar artery may supply the medulla and thus may be damaged with attempts to elevate the cerebellar vermis or by mistake, the medullary kink. Subpial resection of a portion of the cerebellar vermis to help gain access to the fourth ventricle may be less traumatic than continued dissection of the vermis off the underlying medulla. A band-like membrane may lie over the foramen of Magendie and must be widely resected to allow

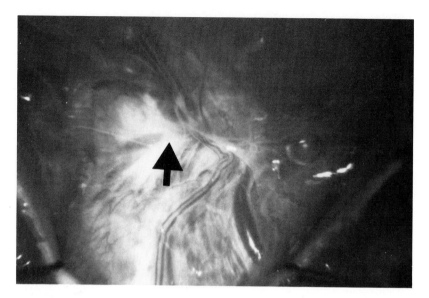

FIGURE 7. Extradural band, syrinx. Intraoperative dorsal view of the cranio-cervical junction of a patient with a Chiari malformation associated with myelodyplasia. Through the intact arachnoid, dense adhesions and vascular constriction under the arch of C1 can be appreciated (arrow).

maximum CSF outflow. Carmel notes that in the process of decompression, itself, grievous errors have resulted from overzealous dissection of tissue.[6] Once access into the fourth ventricle has been obtained, this access can be maintained by the placement of a conduit or stent to ensure continued egress of fluid from the fourth ventricle to the cervical subarachnoid space (Figure 8), a goal enhanced by the placement of a dural graph to expand the subarachnoid space.

For patients with adequately controlled hydrocephalus whose condition progresses despite posterior fossa decompression and who have syringomyelia, other surgical options are available. These basically include procedures directed at removal of fluid from the syrinx rather than preventing its accumulation. Shunt tubes placed inside the syrinx have attempted to divert fluid into the subarachnoid space, the pleural space, and the peritoneum, among other places. These procedures are generally less effective than posterior fossa decompression, but in the selected patient may be beneficial.

VIII. PROGNOSIS

Because of the variable natural history of Chiari-related brain stem signs and symptoms (one third of infants with symptoms die and two thirds remain stable at a compromised level or recover spontaneously), management decisions are complicated.

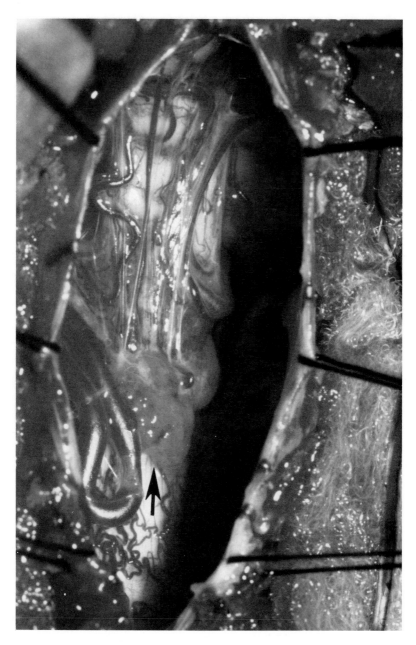

A

FIGURE 8. Photo of stent in place. (A) Intraoperative view of the caudally descended cerebellar vermis (horizontal folli) and the extraventricular choroid plexus (arrow). Immediately to the left of the arrow is the left posterior inferior cerebellar artery. (B) Same patient as A with stent in place, opening the foramen of Magendie and communicating the fourth ventricle with the cervical subarachnoid space.

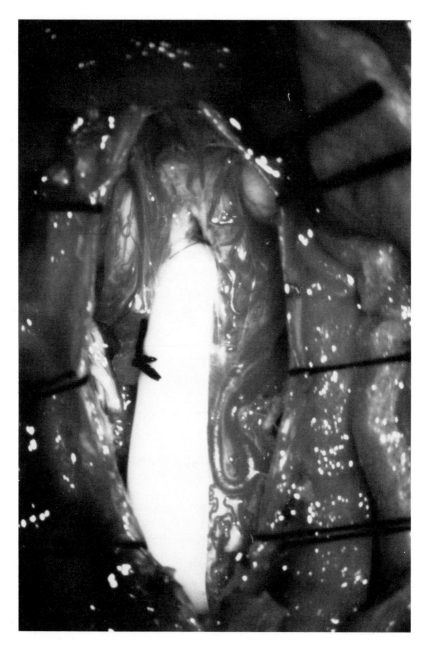

FIGURE 8B.

The more symptoms a child has (stridor, apnea and bradycardia, cyanotic spells, and dysphagia), the more likely it is the child will die of brain stem dysfunction with or without posterior fossa decompression and laminectomy.[36] Infants with the most symptoms presumably have the most abnormal brain stems. Posterior fossa decompression and laminectomy cannot be expected to improve diffuse brain stem infarcts, marked dysmorphology, or absent cranial nerve nuclei. It may improve perfusion, release traction, or equalize pressure. Intraoperative and immediate postoperative mortality and morbidity are low with less than 5% of patients suffering a permanent significant injury as a result of the procedure. Complications include sterile eosinophilic meningitis requiring removal of the stent, bacterial meningitis, painful cervical kyphosis, and damage to the exposed neural tissue from trauma or vascular compromise.

Repeat operations for stent replacement in our series did not relieve additional symptoms. Two patients were unchanged and one deteriorated despite reoperation. In our series and in another,[36] long-term outcome for infants with lower cranial nerve symptoms and signs of sufficient degree to warrant intervention who have posterior fossa decompression and laminectomy is poor, with about one third improved and most of the rest expired.

In contrast, we and others[7,35,49] have had good results for patients with spasticity as their principal reason for surgery. The clear majority were vastly improved at follow-up.

Because of the reversibility of potentially lethal symptoms in some patients and because of the low risks involved in surgery, we feel that posterior fossa decompression and laminectomy is justified in children with serious brain stem symptoms. Improvement in criteria for selection of operative candidates and in the ability to prognosticate based on electrophysiologic testing will help delineate patients into subgroups. This may improve the operative results in some patients and avoid operating on others where the situation is hopeless.

IX. SUMMARY

In summary, the Chiari malformation associated with myelomeningoceles may present a myriad of clinical signs and symptoms depending upon age. Anatomically, the lesion encountered most commonly would be categorized as a type II Chiari malformation. This consists of a wide variety of pathological changes, including caudal displacement of the cerebellar vermis and the lower brain stem through the foramen magnum. Symptoms may present from infancy through adolescence and beyond. Symptoms include lower cranial nerve dysfunction, spasticity, and sensory loss. The Chiari malformations can be explained by a combination of hydrodynamic and pressure gradient theories occurring at different embryologic times. Some component of primary dysgenesis cannot be discounted as a contributing factor. Techniques for evaluation include radiographs of the skull and cervical spine as well as MRI of the brain and cervical spinal cord. The surgical approach, after assuring adequate relief of increased intracranial pressure if present, consists of posterior fossa decompression and laminectomy and the establishment and maintenance of CSF outflow from the fourth ventricle to the cervical subarachnoid space. Although improvement may be seen, a significant number of patients with serious respiratory symptomatology will deteriorate despite surgical intervention. This underscores our limited understanding of the basic mechanisms responsible for hindbrain hernias.

REFERENCES

1. **Aboulezz, A. O., Sartork, B., Geyer, C. A., and Gado, M. H.,** Position of cerebellar tonsils in the normal population and in patients with Chiari malformation: a quantitative approach with MR imaging, *J. Comput. Assist. Tomogr.,* 9, 1033, 1985.
2. **Bell, W. O., Charuey, E. G., Bruce, D. A. et al.,** Symptomatic Arnold-Chiari malformation: review of experience with 22 cases, *J. Neurosurg.,* 66, 812, 1987.
3. **Bluestone, C. B., Delerme, A. N., and Samuelson, G. H.,** Airway obstruction due to vocal cord paralysis in infants with hydrocephalus and meningomyelocele, *Am. Otol.,* 81, 778, 1972.
4. **Cahan, L. D. and Bentson, J. R.,** Considerations in the diagnosis and treatment of syringomyelia and the Chiari malformation, *J. Neurosurg.,* 57, 34, 1982.
5. **Cameron, A. H.,** The Arnold-Chiari and other neuro-anatomical malformations associated with spina bifida, *J. Pathol. Bacteriol.,* 75, 195, 1957.
6. **Carmel, P. W.,** Management of the Chiari malformations in childhood, *Clin. Neurosurg.,* 30, 385, 1983.
7. **Charuey, E. B., Rorke, L. B., Sutton, L. N. et al.,** Management of Chiari II complications in infants with myelomeningocele, *J. Pediatr.,* 111, 364, 1987.
8. **Daniel, P. W. and Strich, S. J.,** Some observations on the congenital deformity of the central nervous system known as the Arnold-Chiari malformation, *J. Neuropathol. Exp. Neurol.,* 17, 255, 1958.
9. **DeLaPaz, R. L., Brady, T. J., Buonanno, F. S. et al.,** Nuclear magnetic resonance imaging of Arnold-Chiari Type I malformation with hydromyelia, *J. Comput. Assist. Tomogr.,* 7, 126, 1983.
10. **DeReuk, J. and VanderEecken, H.,** The arterial angioarchitecture of the Arnold-Chiari malformation, *Arch. Biol.,* 88, 61, 1977.
11. **Emery, J. L.,** Deformity of the aqueduct of Sylvius in children with hydrocephalus and myelomeningocele, *Dev. Med. Child Neurol.,* 16(Suppl. 32), 40, 1974.
12. **Emery, J. L. and Levick, R. K.,** The movement of the brain stem and vessels around the brain stem in children with hydrocephalus and the Arnold-Chiari malformation, *Dev. Med. Child Neurol.,* 16(Suppl. 11), 49, 1966.
13. **Emery, J. L. and MacKenzie, N.,** Medullo-cervical dislocation deformity (Chiari II deformity) related to neurospinal dysraphism (meningomyelocele), *Brain,* 96, 155, 1973.
14. **Faria, M. A., Hoffman, J. C., and O'Brien, M. S.,** Metrizamide cisternography and the management of the Chiari II malformation, *Child's Brain,* 11, 242, 1984.
15. **Gardner, W. J.,** Hydrodynamic mechanism of syringomyelia: its relationship to myelocele, *J. Neurol. Neurosurg. Psychiat.,* 28, 247, 1965.
16. **Gendell, H. M., McCallum, J. E., and Reigel, D. H.,** Cricopharyngeal achloasia associated with Arnold-Chiari malformation in childhood, *Child's Brain,* 4, 65, 1978.

17. **Gilbert, J. N., Jones, K. L., Rorke, L. B. et al.,** Central nervous system anomalies associated with meningomyelocele, hydrocephalus, and the Arnold-Chiari malformation: reappraisal of theories regarding the pathogenesis of posterior neural tube closure defects, *Neurosurgery*, 5, 559, 1986.

18. **Hoffman, H. J., Henrich, E. B., and Humphreys, R. P.,** Manifestations and management of Arnold-Chiari malformation in patients with myelomeningocele, *Child's Brain*, 1, 255, 1975.

19. **Holinger, P. C., Holinger, L. D., Reichert, T. J., and Holinger, P. H.,** Respiratory obstruction and apnea in infants with meningomyocele/hydrocephalus, and Arnold-Chiari malformation, *J. Pediatr.*, 92, 328, 1978.

20. **Holliday, P. O., Pillsbury, D., Kelly, D. L., and Dillard, R.,** Brain stem auditory evoked potentials in Arnold-Chiari malformation: possible prognostic value and changes with surgical decompression, *Neurosurgery*, 16, 48, 1985.

21. **Kirsch, W. M., Duncan, B. R., Black, F. O., and Stears, J. C.,** Laryngeal palsy in association with myelomeningocele, hydrocephalus, and the Arnold-Chiari malformation, *J. Neurosurg.*, 28, 207, 1968.

22. **Lapides, J., Diokno, A. C., Silber, S. J. et al.,** Clean intermittent self-catheterization in the treatment of urinary tract disease, *J. Urol.*, 107, 458, 1972.

23. **Lichtenstein, B. W.,** Distant neuroanatomic complications of spina bifida (spinal dysraphism), *Arch. Neurol. Psychiat.*, 47, 195, 1942.

24. **McLendon, R. E., Crain, B. J., Oakes, W. J., and Burger, P. C.,** Cerebral polygyria in the Chiari Type II (Arnold-Chiari) malformation, *Clin. Neuropathol.*, 4, 200, 1985.

25. **McLone, D. G.,** Results of treatment of children born with a myelomeningocele, *Clin. Neurosurg.*, 30, 407, 1983.

26. **McLone, D. G., Dias, L., Kaplan, W. E., and Sommers, M. W.,** Concepts in the management of spina bifida, *Concepts Pediat. Neurosurg.*, 5, 97, 1985.

27. **Modic, M. T., Weinstein, M. A., Pavlicek, W. et al.,** Magnetic resonance imaging of the cervical spine: technical and clinical observations, *AJR*, 141, 1129, 1983.

28. **Morley, A. R.,** Laryngeal stridor, Arnold-Chiari malformation and medullary hemorrhages, *Dev. Med. Child Neurol.*, 11, 471, 1969.

29. **Naidich, T. P., Pudlowski, R. M., Naidich, J. B. et al.,** Computed tomographic signs of the Chiari malformation. I. Skull and dural partitions, *Neuroradiology*, 134, 391, 1980.

30. **Naidich, T. P., Pudlowski, R. M., and Naidich, J. B.,** Computed tomographic signs of the Chiari II malformation. II. Midbrain and cerebellum, *Neuroradiology*, 134, 391, 1980.

31. **Naidich, T. P., Pudlowski, R. M., and Naidich, J. B.,** Computed tomographic signs of the Chiari malformation. III. Ventricles and cisterns, *Neuroradiology*, 134, 657, 1980.

32. **Naidich, T. P., McLone, D. G., and Fulling, K. H.,** The Chiari II malformation. IV. The hindbrain deformity, *Neuroradiology*, 26, 179, 1983.

33. **Newman, P. K., Terenty, T. R., and Foster, J. B.,** Some observations on the pathogenesis of syringomyelia, *J. Neurol. Neurosurg. Psychiat.*, 44, 964, 1981.

34. **Oakes, W. J.,** Symptomatic Chiari malformation in infant and childhood, *Child's Brain*, 8, 217, 1981.

35. **Oakes, W. J., Worley, G., Spock, A., and Whiting, K.,** Surgical intervention in twenty-nine patients with symptomatic Type II Chiari malformations: clinical presentation and outcome, *Concepts Pediatr. Neurosurg.*, 8, 76, 1988.

36. **Oren, J., Kelly, D. H., Todres, I. D., and Shannon, D. C.,** Respiratory complications in patients with myelodysplasia and Arnold-Chiari malformation, *Am. J. Dis. Child*, 140, 221, 1986.

37. **Osaka, K., Tanimura, T., Hirayama, A., and Matsumoto, S.,** Myelomeningocele before birth, *J. Neurosurg.*, 49, 711, 1978.

38. **Papasozomenos, S. and Roessmann, U.,** Respiratory distress and the Arnold-Chiari malformation, *Neurology (NY)*, 31, 97, 1981.

39. **Park, T. S., Hoffman, H. J., Hendrick, E. B., and Humphreys, R. P.,** Experience with surgical decompression of the Arnold-Chiari malformation in young infants with myelomeningocele, *Neurosurgery,* 13, 147, 1983.

40. **Patten, B. M.,** Overgrowth of neural tube in young human embryos, *Anat. Rec.,* 113, 381, 1952.

41. **Peach, B.,** The Arnold-Chiari malformation: morphogenesis, *Arch. Neurol.,* 12, 527, 1965.

42. **Peach, B.,** Arnold-Chiari malformation. Anatomic features of 20 cases, *Arch. Neurol.,* 12, 613, 1965.

43. **Penfield, W. and Coburn, D. F.,** Arnold-Chiari malformation and its operative treatment, *Arch. Neurol. Psychiat.,* 40, 328, 1938.

44. **Shut, L. and Bruce, D. A.,** The Arnold-Chiari malformation, *Orthoped. Clin. N. Am.,* 9(4), 913, 1978.

45. **Sieben, R. L., Hamida, M. B., and Shulman, K.,** Multiple cranial nerve deficits associated with the Arnold-Chiari malformation, *Neurology,* 21, 675, 1971.

46. **Stone, J. L., Bonfford, A., Morris, R., Dovsepian, W., and Meyers, L. H.,** Clinical and electrophysiologic recovery in Arnold-Chiari malformation, *Surg. Neurol.,* 20, 313, 1983.

47. **Tomita, T. and McLone, D. G.,** Acute respiratory arrest. A complication of malfunction of the shunt in children with myelomeningocele and the Arnold-Chiari malformation, *Am. J. Dis. Child,* 137, 142, 1983.

48. **Venes, J. L.,** Multiple cranial nerve palsies in an infant with the Arnold-Chiari malformation, *Dev. Med. Child Neurol.,* 16, 817, 1974.

49. **Venes, J. L., Black, K. L., and Latack, J. T.,** Preoperative evaluation and surgical management of the Arnold-Chiari malformation, *J. Neurosurg.,* 64, 363, 1986.

50. **Wealthall, S. R., Whittaker, G. E., and Greenwood, N.,** The relationship of apnea and stridor in spina bifida to other unexplained infant deaths, *Dev. Med. Child Neurol.,* 10(suppl. 132), 107, 1974.

51. **Welch, K., Shillito, J., Strand, R. et al.,** Chiari I "malformations" — an acquired disorder, *J. Neurosurg.,* 55, 604, 1981.

52. **Williams, B.,** Chronic herniation of the hindbrain, *Ann. R. Coll. Surg. Engl.,* 63, 9, 1981.

Chapter 5

NEUROSURGICAL MANAGEMENT OF THE CHILD WITH SPINA BIFIDA

Harold L. Rekate

TABLE OF CONTENTS

The potential for late deterioration in children with myelomeningocele creates a burden of responsibility on their caretakers for compulsive follow-up and assessment that is greater than for most of the afflictions of humans and that lasts throughout the length of the child's life. Unless associated with other severe anomalies of brain development, perinatal anoxia, or ventriculitis, children born with myelomeningocele and the Chiari II malformation have a spread of IQ similar to, but slightly lower than, the unaffected population.[1-3] Specific difficulties with various learning tasks, particularly mathematics, is well recognized in children with spina bifida. In a long-term follow-up of a stable spina bifida population, Bartoshesky and colleagues have shown that 85% of children who have been managed aggressively are functioning at grade level, but 61% of these are in special classes, primarily because of their orthopedic handicaps.[4] In a review of the Cincinnati experience, Oppenheimer has shown that success in regular school settings depends on the level of paraplegia: only 50% of children with thoracolumbar lesions were in regular classes, 76% with midlumbar lesions, and 86% with lower level lesions.[5]

Children with hydrocephalus (i.e., who have been shunted) have a slight, but statistically significant, decrease in their IQ scores compared to the small unshunted population.[1] There are, however, many bright and very bright children in both groups. The presence of hydrocephalus, if adequately treated, is entirely consistent with an excellent intellectual outcome.[1-3]

The motor examination in the neonatal period defines the motor potential of the child for the future. While there are reports of improvement in neurologic function following myelomeningocele closure,[6] it must be assumed that the neurologic deficit seen in the newborn period reflects the degree of neurological dysfunction due to the absence of functional neurologic tissue and is, therefore, irrecoverable.[7-10] It also represents the threshold for medical or surgical intervention. If a child is ever noticed to have a lesser level of function than that predicted by the neonatal examination, it must be assumed that some process is causing the deterioration. That process must be aggressively pursued diagnostically and treated promptly. As seen below, deterioration may be from a variety of problems, and it is often impossible to tell whether tethering, syringomyelia, or a symptomatic Chiari malformation has caused the difficulty. In such cases, it is occasionally necessary to treat two or all three conditions at the same time, or in stages. This aggressive posture toward management is most likely to preserve the greatest function and the greatest likelihood of a successful, independent existence for children with spina bifida.

I. HYDROCEPHALUS

In children with spina bifida and the Chiari malformation, hydrocephalus has many features that distinguish it from other forms of hydrocephalus. This is due to the cause of the hydrocephalus as well as to the specific sensitivities of the forebrain, brain stem, and spinal cord to cerebrospinal fluid (CSF) absorptive defects. Caldarelli has shown that in most children with spina bifida, CSF absorption is defective at low pressures and becomes normal as pressures begin to ascend into high ranges.[11] This pop-off phenomenon seems to lead to insidious deterioration in many children at the time of shunt malfunction but protects against overt symptoms of intracranial hypertension in most children with spina bifida.

A. The Concept of Shunt Independence

The question of whether a child, once shunted, can do well without a shunt has been debated in the neurosurgical literature. Views range from that of Holtzer[12] who believes that most children may do without a shunt regardless of the etiology of the hydrocephalus to those of Foltz who states, "Once a shunt, always a shunt."[13] There is little information available from the literature with which to make this decision in the specific case of hydrocephalus associated with the Chiari II malformation. Hall and colleagues first documented the importance of the spinal cord in compensating for hydrocephalus in the Chiari II malformation. They showed that progressive scoliosis was often due to hydromyelia in children with spina bifida who had nonworking shunts and the intracranial symptomatology. Shunt repair often resolved the hydromyelia and improved or stabilized the scoliotic curve. The shunt was needed despite the absence of classical symptoms of shunt malfunction.[14]

The compensation of hydrocephalus at the expense of the spinal cord can be presumed from complications of spine surgery. While unreported in the medical literature, two teenagers suddenly died during surgery for spinal stabilization. In both cases, there had been no shunt revisions for prolonged periods, and no attempt was made to assess shunt functioning preoperatively. In one case at autopsy, the ventricles were enlarged, the shunt was nonfunctional, and evidence of acute intracranial hypertension with herniation was found.[27] In a third case, a child undergoing a resection of a myelokyphosis had a small ventricle and a functioning shunt by preoperative assessment. Intraoperatively, her intracranial pressure (ICP) was measured by a 25-gauge butterfly inserted into the shunt reservoir and connected to a Statham pressure transducer. During spinal instrumentation, ICP rose to 30 torr but responded to pumping of the shunt. After shunt pumping, ICP remained less than 10 torr for the remainder of the operation.[28] Patients with spina bifida undergoing major spinal fusions must have properly functioning shunts before surgery.

A large number of children cared for from birth at Case Western Reserve University in Cleveland were studied for shunt dependency. All patients in the study group of 51 had been proven to have nonworking shunts either by surgical exploration, ligation, or use of an on-off device.[15] Trials of shunt occlusion were never successful in children with noncommunicating hydrocephalus but were successful in 50% (24 of 48) of children with communicating hydrocephalus. These children were shown to not need their shunt, and their intellectual and motor function were just as good after shunt occlusion. In children with spina bifida, however, review of this patient population led to an entirely different result. Twelve children with spina bifida and the Chiari II malformation were occluded or shown to have nonfunctional shunts. Of these, four patients suffered respiratory arrest 18 h to 5 years after occlusion. None of these children had recognized warning signs of intracranial hypertension. Two children died. Two underwent resuscitation and shunt reinsertion and were left with severe intellectual and motor impairments.[15] Other authors have recognized the syndrome of sudden death in children with spina bifida and have thought that it was related to the abnormal relationships of the brain stem within the cervical spinal canal.[16] Once children are shunted for hydrocephalus in the context of spina bifida, they *must* be assumed to be shunt-dependent for life.[17]

B. Insidious Shunt Malfunction

Unique to the context of spina bifida and the Chiari II malformation, shunt malfunction may be insidious with extremely subtle signs and symptoms. The relationship of shunt malfunction to spinal cord damage and scoliosis has been discussed above. In the author's experience, the most common first sign of shunt malfunction in the older child and adolescent with spina bifida is staring spells similar to *absence* attacks. The parents relate that the child will stop talking in the middle of a sentence and stare into space. These spells last only a few seconds to a minute and can be aborted by stimuli such as loud noises or gentle shaking. Because this symptom is not listed in the standard brochures on shunts and not recognized by all caretakers, it is often thought to be behavioral or suggestive of a seizure disorder. Often, these signs do not lead to neurosurgical referral, and the child is not seen until overt signs of seizure, headache, vomiting, and lethargy occur. Computed tomography (CT) or magnetic resonance imaging (MRI) at this point will show enlarged ventricles (Figure 1). A retrospective review will often show a history of months or even years of decline in school performance and attention. Shunt revision will lead to resolution of staring spells and other symptoms, decrease in ventricular size, and often rapid improvement in school performance.

Staring spells in shunted children with spina bifida probably indicate that the shunt is not working and must be repaired.

II. THE TETHERED SPINAL CORD

The name, tethered spinal cord, implies that the spinal cord is attached tightly to a congenitally abnormal structure in the lumbosacral area as well as being attached to the brain at the craniovertebral junction. As the child grows, the spinal cord is stretched between these two points, and neurologic deterioration may result. Originally, it was thought that patients deteriorate during rapid growth spurts, but more recently it has been shown that a child will most likely deteriorate at a time of relatively slow-growth velocity (6.5 years).[18]

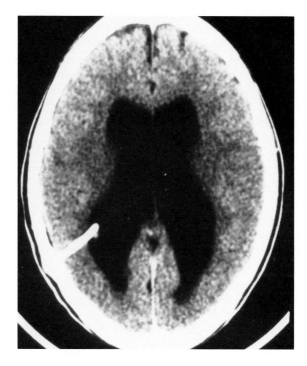

FIGURE 1. CT scan of child with spina bifida whose only complaint was of "staring spells". A subsequent history revealed a significant decline in school performance. The scan shows greater significant ventriculomegaly.

Yamada has shown that the mechanical stretching of the cord during physical activity leads to changes in intracellular respiration as shown by studies of cytochrome oxidase and proposes this as a cause of neurologic deterioration in the tethered-cord syndrome.[19]

The tethered-cord syndrome may be from a number of congenital anomalies, including thickening of the filum terminale, intraspinal lipoma, diastematomyelia, and a variety of other "occult" dysraphic states.[20] In this discussion, tethered cord refers to the scarring of the neural placode or spinal cord to the overlying dura or skin at the site of myelomeningocele repair. With new imaging modalities, particularly MRI, it is apparent that tethering as an anatomic entity is present in virtually all children who have undergone myelomeningocele closure, regardless of lesion level or method of repair.

While the presence of a low, posteriorly affixed conus medullaris on neuroimaging studies in occult dysraphism is, in and of itself, a clear indication for surgical detethering, indications for detethering the child with spina bifida cystica remain controversial. Few would recommend detethering all children with anatomically tethered cords who have no overt symptoms. However, as experience grows, this view may begin to predominate. Most pediatric neurosurgeons will intervene to detether a spinal cord in spina bifida children once even subtle signs of neurologic deterioration are detected.

Recognized signs of symptomatic tethered cord include back and leg pain, change in bladder tone, incontinence on intermittent catheter, change in motor or sensory level in the lower extremities, spasticity, and, most controversial of all, scoliosis.

A representative case illustrates the typical presentation of a child with spina bifida and a symptomatic tethered cord.

> RR, a 9.5-year-old-male, was born with a lower sacral myelomeningocele. He underwent closure of the myelomeningocele defect in the second day of life and was shunted during that hospitalization. Neurologic examination performed 3 months before his hospitalization revealed a functioning shunt, no cranial deficits, and normal motor funtion of the upper and lower extremities. Sensory examination revealed a lack of bilateral perianal and penile sensation, and there was no anal wink. He was on clean intermittent catheterization (CIC) every 4 to 6 h and was dry between catheterizations. About 6 weeks before his hospitalization, he rapidly lost urinary continence despite catheterization every 2 h and was required to wear diapers for the first time in 4 years. Four weeks before admission he began experiencing vague pains in his lower back and a burning numbness in his feet. MRI revealed his spinal cord to be plastered against the back of the spine and to be bent outward abruptly at the S1 level of intact lamina to end in a subcutaneous scar (Figure 2). The child underwent a detethering operation as described below. His back pain and feet numbness completely resolved within the first few days of surgery. By 6 weeks, the child was again continent on CIC every 4 h but with the addition of ditropan to increase bladder capacity.

A. Development of Tethered-Cord Syndrome in Children with Spina Bifida

The potential for development of the tethered-cord syndrome essentially begins with the closure of the myelomeningocele defect. As described, the techniques of closure of the original myelomeningocele defect represent an attempt to prevent the secondary tethering caused by scarring. The neural placode is inverted into a tube preventing contact with the overlying dura of subcutaneous tissue. Afterward, a watertight dural closure is essential but should be loose to maintain a reservoir of CSF around this newly formed tubular structure, allowing the spinal cord to float freely and not be restricted in a compartment to which it could become attached.

While these suggestions for closure are logical, there is no evidence that they prevent tethering. Essentially, all sagittal MRIs of the spines of children with spina bifida seem to show tethering, with the spinal cord adhering to the area of repair. Despite the surgical techniques to prevent tethering, there may be anatomic reasons why it is inevitable in these children. Figure 3 shows the change in orientation of the spine and spinal cord as the child grows. The area

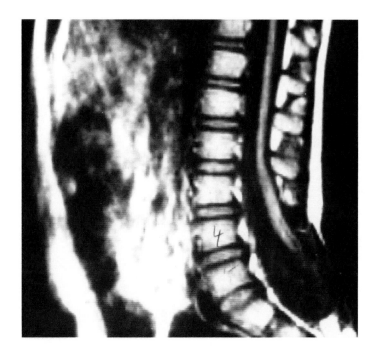

FIGURE 2. MRI scan of child with a lumbosacral level myelomeningocele demonstrating tethering of the spinal cord.

of the intraspinal compartment is very shallow, like a dish. With closure of the myelomeningocele, the shallow dish is covered by dura and overlying soft tissue; however, when the child lies on his or her back, the spinal cord remnant must be compressed in this envelope. As the child grows (Figure 3, bottom), the physical dimensions of the spine increase. The child also develops a lumbar lordosis associated with bipedal gait. This lumbar lordosis is often accentuated in spina bifida. The result of these two phenomema is the conversion of a spinal plate into a fluted glass. The spinal cord, which is now attached to the overlying dura and scar, becomes bent around the last intact lamina to attach to the scar of the back at right angles. This dorsally affixed spinal cord is uniformly found in association with a copious CSF-containing compartment anterior to the spinal cord. This fluted glass arrangement is a much more convenient anatomic compartment to prevent tethering than the shallow dish of infancy.

B. Signs and Symptoms of Symptomatic Tethered Cord

Selection of patients with spina bifida who should undergo detethering procedures is controversial and, to some extent, is in a state of flux as the early and late results of treatment begin to be reported. Despite the complexity and individual variation in anatomy of these patients, risks for decreased neurologic function from surgery appear to be low and improvements in neurologic

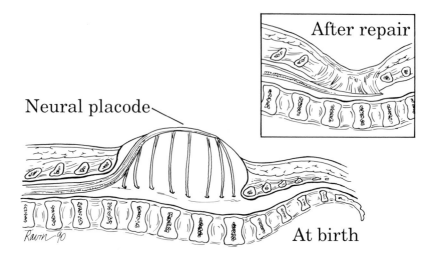

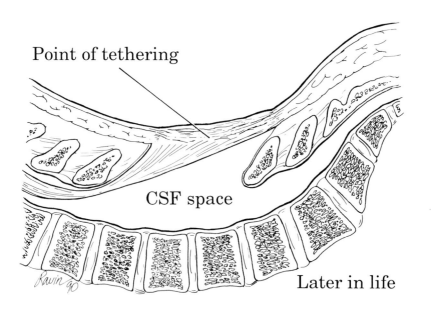

FIGURE 3. Tethering of the spinal cord in spina bifida. (Top) In the newborn the spinal canal is very shallow, and the repair is covered by an envelope of dura and skin in a small space. (Bottom) As the child grows and develops the normal lumbar lordosis, the canal assumes a fluted-glass appearance. When the spinal cord is detethered, it drops by gravity into the canal and allows CSF to flow around it, hopefully preventing retethering.

function frequent. This leads to a progressive lowering of the threshold for recommending surgical management of tethered cord in spina bifida patients.

Loss of neurologic function in the lower extremities represents the most compelling as well as the most urgent indication for detethering the spinal cord. This deterioration can either be loss of lower motor neuron function above the previous lesion level or increasing difficulties with gait as a result of spasticity. Spasticity presents in two distinct ways. As in children with spasticity from other causes, the increased tone leads to increased energy requirements in movements of the lower extremities and makes movements slower and more difficult. In the specific context of spina bifida, there are often muscle imbalances due to the lesion level. When spasticity is also present, the potential exists for the involved joint to become deformed and not to respond as expected to orthopedic procedures. In children with midlumbar myelomeningoceles, hip flexors are present, but functional hip extension is lost. This leads to the strong likelihood of flexion-contractions or subluxation at this point. If spasticity is present in the iliopsoas musculature, this problem is accentuated. Recurrent subluxation or contractions after orthopedic stabilization of the hip may mean spasticity, and in this context, tethering, unless another cause is found.

Pain is a variable feature of spinal-cord tethering in patients with spina bifida. Pain as a symptom of spinal-cord tethering can be localized to the back or can have a radicular character. Pain is not present in all patients with overtly symptomatic spinal-cord tethering. Pain limited to the lower back is difficult to assess. Spinal deformities and accentuation of lumbar lordosis, which are common in context of spina bifida, may lead to back pain without involving spinal-cord tethering. Currently, severe and functionally limiting lower back pain as a symptom may be used to support the diagnosis of spinal-cord tethering, but rarely is it the only symptom leading to surgical repair. Radicular pain, however, is strongly linked to spinal-cord tethering. Bilateral leg pain is an especially strong indication for surgical intervention.

Deterioration in bladder function is the most common indication for surgical intervention in the context of spina bifida and supports the importance of caring for children with spina bifida in multidisciplinary clinics. It is the urologist who will first be made aware of difficulties when children who were previously continent on CIC begin to have accidents and require catheterization more frequently. Urinary continence is extremely important for the child's socialization and eventually for his or her potential for acceptance as an independent organism. Its loss is a serious blow. Detethering will lead to a larger capacity bladder, longer intervals between catheterization, and a better chance to stay dry. We have found that some children who have never achieved continence on CIC have succeeded after detetherings have been performed for other reasons.

As a sign of spinal-cord tethering, scoliosis is the subject of much debate. Scoliosis is common in the context of spina bifida and has a variety of causes.

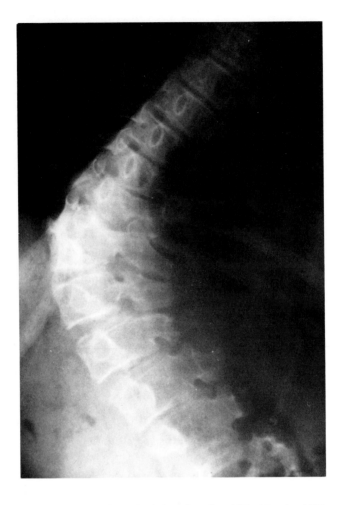

FIGURE 4. Plain radiograph of the spine of a child with spina bifida showing scoliosis secondary to hemivertebrae.

Bony anomalies, such as hemivertebrae of the spine and multiple rib fusion, may lead inevitably to scoliosis, independent of neurologic functioning (Figure 4). Also, the anatomic lesion level may be different on one side than on the other and lead to imbalances in the paravertebral musculature, thereby resulting in scoliosis. In the absence of these predisposing factors, however, scoliosis should be preventable in most spina bifida children. When progressive, scoliosis often means that changes are occurring in the segmental innervation of the paravertebral musculature. Clearly, these changes can be from syringomyelia, which is related to hydrocephalus and shunt function, and are discussed below. Without the predisposing causes described above, scoliosis will likely develop from tethering. If progressive scoliosis is noted by orthopedics, detethering should be performed before the curve becomes self-perpetuating. As a corollary, if a child with severe scoliosis is documented to have tethering on an imaging study and if treatment of the scoliosis involves significant spinal straightening, the spinal cord should be detethered prophylactically to prevent damage to the spinal cord during surgery.

C. Surgical Principles

The anatomic details of the relationship of the spinal cord to surrounding structures differ in each child, and these differences may not be obvious from imaging studies. Following simple surgical principles should lead to successful repair in most cases. There are two goals of surgery for tethered cord in the context of myelomeningocele: (1) release of the spinal cord/neural placode from its attachments to the overlaying scar and (2) creation of a watertight dural closure to form a large reservoir of CSF to surround the released cord and to prevent retethering.

Based on midsagittal MRIs (Figure 2), the spinal cord is usually seen to dead end onto the skin-covered neural placode. The space anterior to the spinal cord at the level of tethering is uniformly found to be copius. Occasionally, the spinal cord is tethered to the overlying skin over a long segment (Figure 5), making the dissection tedious and more dangerous. The first step in performing a detethering operation, when possible, is to identify the last intact spinous process above the neural placode. When this is removed, previously undisturbed dura can be identified. Epidural fat and ligamentum flavum are removed, and extradural dissection is carried caudally until the scar where the dura and skin are sealed together can be identified. The flared laminae are then seen to spread outward, and a subperiosteal dissection is carried laterally on both sides. Some inwardly pointing laminar elements may need to be removed for exposure.

At this point, the dura is opened and the intradural exploration performed under the operating microscope. We have most commonly found that an upwardly cutting #12 blade can be invaluable in the dural opening as the dura, neural placode, and skin begin to fuse. Just proximal to the point of fusion, the dorsal root entry zone is identified. This identification is crucial since dissection dorsal to the dorsal root entry zone should allow detethering to proceed without harming the functioning neural elements. Occasionally, it appears as if the nerve roots themselves are the tethering elements; however, there is ususally an investing and occasionally dense adhesive arachnoiditis enveloping the roots that can be dissected to free the spinal cord.

Dissection then proceeds caudally above the dorsal root entry zone until the entire neural placode and spinal cord fall into the hole created by the copious anterior spinal subarachnoid space. This "falling" of the spinal cord heralds the successful completion of the detethering process; however, the relationship of the neural placode, scar, and nerve roots should be explored thoroughly. Occasionally, skin elements are inverted into the closure at the time of primary

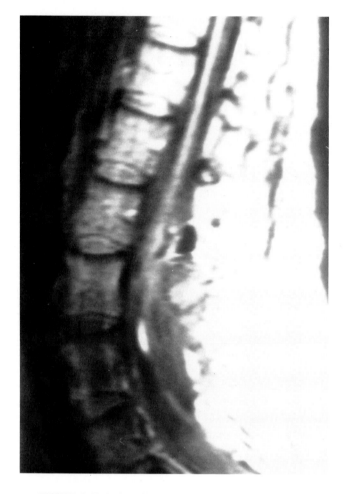

FIGURE 5. Tethering of the spinal cord over a long segment.

repair and create a dermoid at the repair site. Should a dermoid be present, it should be removed as a potential source of retethering.

Closure of the repair is critical to the success of the operation. After the scar tissue is removed from the dural edges, primary repair is frequently, if not uniformly, difficult. Also, one of the essential surgical principles is that a watertight dural closure allowing a copious amount of CSF to surround the neural placode should be made. If the dural repair is at all snug, retethering becomes inevitable. Dural grafting with lyophilized cadaver dura or autologous fascia lata in a watertight fashion is uniformly required. A Valsalva maneuver is performed to assure watertight closure prior to fascial and skin closure. In the upper lumbar and thoracic regions, fascial closure can be performed with dissectiom and undermining. In the lumbosacral region, this is often impossible and one must rely on the dural closure and skin closure only.

After an operation to detether the spinal cord, the patient is nursed, if tolerated, in a prone position for about 3 d to keep the spinal cord away from the dural repair. Postoperatively, MRIs taken in the standard supine position rarely show changes from the preoperative scans, except for the absence of the most caudal intact spinous process despite almost uniform improvement in the patient's preoperative condition. Because of movement artifacts from breathing, MRI in the prone position is difficult to perform and interpret. When properly gaited, however, these images can show the presence of CSF posterior to the neural placode, thereby confirming adequate detethering.

Secondary tethering of the neural placode, resulting in further deterioration in neurologic function, is said to occur in 10 to 15% of patients undergoing detethering operations, regardless of the techniques used. Radiographic diagnosis of retethering is extremely difficult to distinguish from normal postoperative changes. The decision to reexplore a child who has undergone a detethering operation must, for the most part, be made entirely on clinical grounds. Several authors have described a technique for the imaging of the spinal cord ultrasonographically through the neural placode. In patients without symptomatic tethering, the spinal cord oscillates with respiratory and cardiac pulsations, and these oscillations can be visualized on real-time ultrasound.[21-24] When tethering occurs, the oscillations are absent or can be completely obliterated with forward flexion of the head. More data are needed about the usefulness of this procedure, however.

III. SYRINGOMYELIA

Syringomyelia is a common finding on MRI in children with spina bifida. Attention to this important condition was first focused by the work of Hall and colleagues,[14] who showed that progressive scoliosis in children with spina bifida was often from syringomyelia. They pointed out that hydrocephalus in the context of spina bifida could become compensated for by the forcing of CSF into the central canal. They showed that performing or reconstituting a shunt would often stabilize or improve scoliotic curves.

Syringomyelia can cause deterioration in neurologic function and can take a variety of forms. Probably the most common is the development of spasticity in patients who should only have lower motor neuron abnormalities. Because of the intrinsic muscular imbalances around each joint in the lower extremities, spasticity may present subtly as a progressive deformity of the knee or hip. Often, normally active reflexes will become more brisk.

Syringomyelia may extend above the brachial plexus outflow and therefore lead to both motor and sensory deterioration in arm function. We have most commonly found moderate to severe syringomyelia in the context of a screening MRI. When this occurs, a careful neurologic examination and history are necessary to ascertain the relationship of current to past neurologic function. Like tethering and the Arnold-Chiari malformation, syringomyelia may lead to insidious deterioration in neurologic function. In a child who is suffering from slow progressive deterioration, it is often impossible to discern which of the pathologies is the cause, and two or all of these must be treated at the same operation. It has been relatively frequent in our experience to encounter a child with the whole spectrum of scoliosis, deterioration in motor function, and deterioration in bladder function requiring a detethering and syringopleural shunt in the same operation.

Syringomyelia is hydrocephalus of the spinal cord and results from high pressure of CSF within the central canal of the spinal cord. The circulation of CSF in the context of the Arnold-Chiari malformation is complex and discussed in detail above. Briefly, however, the intracranial compartment is isolated from the spinal CSF compartment. In untreated hydrocephalus, either from a shunt never having been installed or in the context of insidious shunt malfunction, CSF that cannot exit the fourth ventricular foramina is forced into the central canal, which distends at the expense of the spinal cord. In these situations, shunting of the ventricles will often reverse the condition. One half of CSF is formed extrachoroidally as extracellular fluid (ECF). Syringomyelia can develop despite small ventricles and working shunts if the CSF within the spinal cord cannot be absorbed either to the shunting mechanism or to the sagittal sinus.

Treatment of syringomyelia in the context of spina bifida by syringosubarachnoid shunt, which is so frequently successful in syringomyelia from other causes, is uniformly unsuccessful in this condition. It fails because the CSF in the spinal subarachnoid space cannot circulate easily to its point of absorption because of the crowding of the cervicomedullary junction. CSF must be vented to an absorption cavity. Because of the low volumes of CSF profused within the syrinx, we advocate syringopleural shunts using the Edwards syringoperitoneal "T" shunt. The pleural cavity is well within the operative field. In our experience, this form of treatment has been uniformly successful. The use of the prone position and syringopleural shunting makes it possible to include the treatment of the syringomyelia and the detethering procedure in the same operative field.

The treatment of syringomyelia by blocking off the obex with a plug of cervical muscle has been shown to be successful in the management of syringomyelia. To plug the obex, one must decompress the Chiari II malformation, and this may add to the efficacy of the procedure. Plugging the obex does not deal with the spinal cord ECF and is not uniformly successful. Several anatomic points are essential to the safe performance of an obex plug in the context of the Chiari II malformation. The first point is that the torcula is frequently found at the level of the foramen magnum in this condition, and the dura should only be opened in the cervical canal. Second, the occluded foramen of Magendie is present well down in the cervical canal (at least C2). It is found by dissecting the dense overlying arachnoid in the cervical region, identifying the choroid plexus, and following it cephalad into the fourth ventricle. It is often necessary to remove the most caudal portion of the cerebellar vermis to accomplish this. The obex is oriented directly perpendicular to the floor of the fourth ventricle at this location. Our current recommendation is that an obex plug be reserved for patients in whom syringopleural shunts have failed to correct the abnormality.

IV. OTHER TREATABLE CAUSES OF DETERIORATION IN THE SPINES OF CHILDREN WITH SPINA BIFIDA

The routine use of MRI for screening children with spina bifida has resulted in finding previously unrecognized pathologies, including spinal-cord compression from arachnoid cysts and diastematomyelia. These abnormalities are often the cause of children not reaching their expected motor developmental potential. They should therefore be dealt with even if it seems to be prophylactic. When dorsal, the cysts should be managed by dissection and resection. They may be present anteriorly in some cases (Figure 6) and may be quite challenging to manage. In these situations, shunting of the cysts to the pleura is required.

Diastematomyelia has shown to be a uniformly progressive disease when it is an isolated finding.[18,25] There is no reason to presume that it would act more benignly in the context of the child with spina bifida. If diastematomyelia is found on screening studies of children with spina bifida who have important level extremity function (lumbar level extremity lesions and below), it should be treated surgically. Surgical management of diastematomyelia requires removal of the bony spur, lysis of the strands connecting the medial spinal cord to the medial dura, and dural closure that incorporates both halves of the spinal cord. This should probably be performed at the same time as a standard detethering of the cord from the neural placode.

V. EVALUATION OF THE CHILD WITH SPINA BIFIDA NEWLY PRESENTING FOR CARE

The first visit with a child with spina bifida and his or her family is a responsibility and an opportunity for all concerned. The child already has a long history of treatment for a complicated problem that must be understood before embarking on new therapies. One, however, must not assume that because the child has no overt symptoms that the child does not need intervention. A child with spina bifida who moves frequently, for example, a military dependent, could deteriorate minimally between each move, because the child has not received continuous care from the same examiner, these small changes may go unrecognized and lead to a subtle decline in functional performance. Not only does the old record need to be reviewed, but an attempt should be made to mentally return the child to the perinatal examination and newly assess what the likely biologic functional capacity should be to determine whether

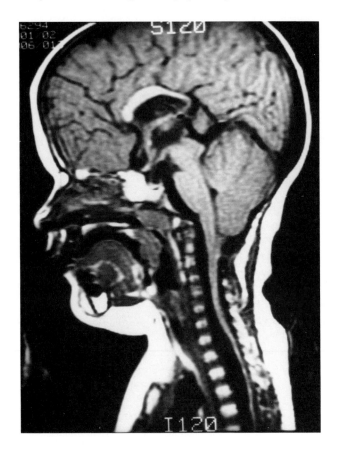

FIGURE 6. MRI showing an arachnoid cyst anterior to the spinal cord, which led to thinning of the cord and neurological deterioration.

any deterioration has occurred. Figure 7 is an algorithm that should prove useful in assessing the older child with spina bifida who is a new patient. Ideally, this neurosurgical assessment should be done in the context of a multidisciplinary team. After the history and neurological examination are performed and available records have been received, three studies should be ordered unless recent studies are available: a shunt series, imaging study of the head (CT or MRI), and an MRI series of the total spine. As has been stated and argued previously, shunt independence is unlikely in the context of spina bifida, and the most pressing issue is that of shunt function. An MRI or CT scan of the head that shows more than mild hydrocephalus should be taken to indicate that the shunt is not working and is needed and should be repaired. Only in the context of very mild ventriculomegaly in a child performing well at school and without significant scoliosis is it justified to "observe" a child with hydrocephalus and spina bifida.[26] If the ventricles are normal or smaller than normal, the shunt is working and should be presumed to be needed.

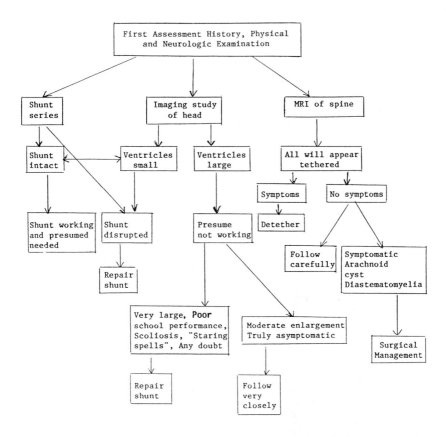

FIGURE 7. Algorithm for assessing the older child who presents to the pediatric neurosurgeon for the first time.

The shunt series is needed to test the length of the shunt and physical integrity of the shunt system. If the shunt is short or apparently disconnected, the shunt should be repaired. The only exception is in the compulsively assessed patient with mild ventriculomegaly who is truly asymptomatic. If there is any doubt about any of these issues, the shunt should be explored and repaired.

An MRI study of the total spine is essential as a screen for children with spina bifida. In all these children, the cord will be said to be tethered anatomically. Eventually, as we learn more about the pathophysiology of tethering as it relates to spina bifida, we may advocate prophylactic detethering of all children with spina bifida. As of now, however, only symptomatic patients from incontinence on CIC, deteriorating motor function, or scoliosis are candidates for detethering.

The other, rarer abnormalities on MRI, including syringomyelia, arachnoid cysts, and diastematomyelia, may be indications for surgical intervention, mostly by their presence on the imaging studies.

After this initial intense reassessment is completed, the child should be followed closely with annual evaluations. As stated above, whenever a child with spina bifida is failing to meet his or her expected functional outcome, it is probably from a treatable condition that must be sought with energy and treated aggressively to optimize the child's potential for a functional, independent life as an adult.

REFERENCES

1. **Mapstone, T. B., Rekate, H. L., Nulsen, F. E., Dixon, M. S., Jr., Glaser, N., and Jaffe, M.,** Relationship of CSF shunting and IQ in children with myelomeningocele: a retrospective analysis, *Child's Brain*, 11, 112, 1984.
2. **McLone, D. G., Czyzewski, D., Raimondi, A. J., and Sommers, R. C.,** Central nervous system infections as a limiting factor in the intelligence of children with myelomeningocele, *Pediatrics*, 70, 338, 1982.
3. **McLone, D. G., Killion, M., Yogev, R., and Sommers, M. W.,** Ventriculitis of mice and men, in *Concepts in Pediatrics Neurosurgery*, Vol. 2, Epstein, F. and Raimondi, A., Eds., S. Karger, Basel, 1982, 112.
4. **Barthoshesky, L. E., Young, G. J., and Scott, R. M.,** Outcomes of children with myelomeningocele treated aggresively from birth, in *Spina Bifida: A Multidisciplinary Approach*, McLaurin, R. L., Oppenheimer, S., Dias, L., and Kaplan, W. E., Eds., Praeger, New York, 1986, 14.
5. **Oppenheimer, S.,** Twenty-year review: Cincinnati experience, in *Spina Bifida: A Multidisciplinary Approach*, McLaurin, R. L., Oppenheimer, S., Dias, L., and Kaplan, W. E., Eds., Praeger, New York, 1986, 8.
6. **Sharrad, W. J. W., Zachery, R. B., Lorber, J. and Bruce, A. M.,** A controlled trial of immediate and delayed closure of spina bifida cystica, *Arch. Dis. Child*, 38, 18, 1963.
7. **Brocklehurst, G., Gleave, J. R. W., and Lewin, W.,** Early closure of myelomeningocele, with special reference to leg movement, *Br. Med. J.*, 1, 666, 1967.
8. **Smyth, B. T., Piggott, J., Forsythe, W. I., and Merrett, J. D.,** A controlled trial of immediate and delayed closure of myelomeningocele, *J. Bone Joint Surg.*, 56B, 297, 1974.
9. **Guthkelch, A. N.,** Thoughts on the surgical management of spina bifida cystica, *Acta Neurochir. (Wein)*, 13, 407, 1965.
10. **Guthkelch, A. N.,** Studies in spina bifida cystica. II. When to repair the spinal defect, *J. Neurol. Neurosurg. Psychiat.*, 25, 137, 1962.
11. **Caldarelli, M., Di Rocco, C., and Rossi, G. F.,** Lumbar subarachnoid infusion test in paediatric neurosurgery, *Dev. Med. Child Neurol.*, 21, 71, 1979.
12. **Holtzer, G. J., and de Lange, S. A.,** Shunt-independent arrest of hydrocephalus, *J. Neurosurg.*, 39, 698, 1973.
13. **Foltz, E. L.,** The first seven years of a hydrocephalus project, in *Workshop in Hydrocephalus*, Shulman, D., Ed., The Children's Hospital of Philadelphia, Philadelphia, 1965, 79.
14. **Hall, P., Lindseth, R., Campbell, R., Kalsbeck, J. E., and Desousa, A.,** Scoliosis and hydrocephalus in myelocele patients. The effects of ventricular shunting, *J. Neurosurg.*, 50, 174, 1979.
15. **Rekate, H. L., Nulsen, F. E., Mack, H. L., and Morrison, G.,** Establishing the diagnosis of shunt independence, *Monogr. Neural Sci.*, 8, 223, 1982.

16. **Staal, M. J., Meihuizen-de Regt, M. J., and Hess, J.,** Sudden death in hydrocephalic spina bifida aperta patients, *Pediatr. Neurosci.,* 13, 13, 1987.

17. **Rekate, H. L.,** Management of hydrocephalus and the erroneous concept of shunt independence in spina bifida patients, *BNI Q.,* 4(4), 17, 1988.

18. **Humphreys, R. P., Hendrick, E. B., and Hoffman, H. J.,** Diastematomyelia, *Clin. Neurosurg.,* 30, 436, 1982.

19. **Yamada, S., Zinke, D. E., and Sanders, D.,** Pathophysiology of "tethered cord syndrome", *J. Neurosurg.,* 54, 494, 1981.

20. **Guthkelch, A. N.,** Occult spinal dysraphism: clinical findings and management, *BNI Q.,* 4(4), 21, 1988.

21. **Di Pietro, M. A. and Venes, J. L.,** Real-time sonography of the pediatric spinal cord: horizons and limits, in *Concepts in Pediatric Neurosurgery,* Vol. 8, Marlin, A. E., Ed., S. Karger, Basel, 1988, 120.

22. **Naidich, T. P., Fernbach, S. K., McLone, D. G., and Shkolnik, A.,** John Caffey Award. Sonography of the caudal spine and back: congenital anomalies in children, *AJR,* 142, 1229, 1984.

23. **Naidich, T. P., McLone, D. G., Shkolnik, A., and Fernbach, S. K.,** Sonographic evaluation of caudal spine anomalies in children, *AJNR,* 4, 661, 1983.

24. **Naidich, T. P., Radkowski, M. A., and Britton, J.,** Real-time sonographic display of caudal spine anomalies, *Neuroradiology,* 28, 512, 1986.

25. **Gutkelch, A. N.,** Diastematomyelia with median septum, *Brain,* 97, 729, 1974.

26. **Rekate, H. L.,** To shunt or not to shunt: hydrocephalus and dysraphism, *Clin. Neurosurg.,* 32, 593, 1985.

27. **Rekate, H. L.,** unpublished data.

28. **Mayfield, J.,** personal communication.

Chapter 6

COMPREHENSIVE ORTHOPEDIC MANAGEMENT IN MYELOMENINGOCELE

Jack K. Mayfield

TABLE OF CONTENTS

I. INTRODUCTION

In general the incidence of myelomeningocele is 1/1000 live births.[123] The incidence is increased in firstborn infants of young mothers and late-born infants of older mothers. In Western Europe, the incidence has been reported at 1.5 to 3/1000 births[15,94] and in Australia the incidence is listed at 0.95/1000 births.[109] Approximately 60% of myelomeningocele patients are female.[40,77] The mortality rate is the highest during infancy with most deaths occurring by 2 years of age.[77] Menelaus has indicated that if a child reaches age 1 year, death is unlikely and active orthopedic treatment is indicated.[77]

The mode of inheritance of spinal dysraphism appears to be multifactorial. There is considerable risk of additional children afflicted with this disorder in the family with one child with an existing neural tube defect. The risk is 1 in 20 for subsequent pregnancies and if two children in a family have neural tube defect, the risk of an additional child with this defect becomes 1 in 2.[53] In this regard it is now possible to make a prenatal diagnosis of neural tube defect in a fetus by assay of α-fetoprotein in the amniotic fluid.[10] Normally this should remain at low levels after 14 weeks of gestation but remain high after 16 weeks of gestation in conditions of neural tube defects. Genetic counseling and prenatal diagnosis are an important aspect of the management of myelomeningocele.

II. NATURAL HISTORY

Lorber noted that the majority of untreated myelodysplastic infants die within 6 months of birth.[61] In untreated patients, death in the first 2 years of life usually results from hydrocephalus or intracranial infection.[54,55] Should an untreated infant survive for 2 months, there is a 28% possibility that he will live to be 7 years of age.[23] A total of 80% of children without hydrocephalus and 50% with hydrocephalus have intelligence quotients above 80.[62] Lorber in a comprehensive evaluation of treated children found that 1/3 of children were ambulators without orthotic assistance, 20% were therapy ambulators, and 1/3 were in wheelchairs full time.[62] In addition, he also found that only 7% of children could compete intellectually with their peers. He found that even though 20% had normal intelligence, the physical handicaps required a sheltered working environment.[62]

III. SELECTION FOR TREATMENT

Spina bifida is a disease with multiple degrees of severity and in the neonatal period, difficult decisions need to be made concerning treatment. Many authors have addressed the desirability and feasibility of treatment.[37,49,61,111–113]

Menelaus, at the Royal Children's Hospital in Melbourne, has indicated that the following features are regarded as contraindications for early sac closure:[77,111]

1. Infected sac at presentation
2. High neurosegmental lesions, especially with kyphosis
3. Hydrocephalus at birth
4. Meningitis
5. Multiple congenital anomalies or other life-threatening diseases

It is Menelaus' opinion that active treatment should begin only if the baby with any of the above conditions survives.

Lorber[61,62] also correlated certain physical findings that related to poor prognosis for survival:

1. Paralysis above L3
2. Congenital rigid kyphosis or scoliosis
3. A grossly enlarged head with a maximum circumference of 2 cm or more above the 90th percentile related to birth weight
4. Intracerebral birth injuries
5. Other gross congenital defects

Furthermore, Lorber indicated that children who develop meningitis or ventriculitis after sac closure should not be treated.[61,62] It was his opinion that active multidisciplinary treatment should be instituted only if the child survives at least 6 months and continues to thrive.[61,62]

The orthopedic surgeon usually is minimally involved in the neonatal period. The only orthopedic condition requiring active treatment in the neonatal period is talipes equinovarus. Since the case mortality is high during the first year of life, further active orthopedic treatment should be delayed until orthopedic assessment at 6 to 12 months of age.[77]

IV. PATHOPHYSIOLOGY

There are several factors that produce limb deformity, abnormal posture, and gait:[77]

1. Muscle imbalance secondary to neurological abnormality
2. Habitually assumed intrauterine posture
3. Habitually assumed posture after birth
4. Coexistent congenital malformations
5. Arthrogryposis
6. Tethering of neural tissue
7. Sensory, cerebral, cerebellar, and upper limb abnormalities
8. Leg-length discrepancy in association with unilateral paralysis

The basic spinal cord lesion in myelomeningocele is not fully understood but it has become apparent that this is not just myelodysplasia with a lower motor neuron deficit. Many children also have upper motor neuron lesions. Many authors have noted upper motor neuron deficits with preserved isolated cord segments distally.[14,22,73,114]

Clinical evidence of upper motor neuron activity is found in 66.6% of children with myelomeningocele.[114] The neurological lesion in spina bifida has been classified by Stark and Baker into two types:[114]

1. Type I lesions: infants with type I lesions have normal function down to a particular level below which there is flaccid paralysis, loss of sensation, and loss of reflexes
2. Type II (a) lesions: infants in this category have a gap in cord function (with loss of motor sensory and reflex activity) and distal to this intact but isolated cord segments
3. Type II (b) lesions: children in this category have a narrow gap in cord function and resemble patients with spinal cord transection; a slight stimulation at any point of the leg generally evokes a flexion withdrawal reflex
4. Type II (c) lesions: there is incomplete cord transection so that the child

has spastic paraplegia but incomplete loss of voluntary movements and sensation[114]

In reviewing 100 consecutive infants with myelomeningocele examined after 24 h of age, Stark found the following neurological pattern:[114]

Normal	8%
Type I	28%
Type II(a)	37%
Type II(b)	18%
Type II(c)	9%

The majority of patients had upper motor neuron lesions and it was concluded that some of the normal and type I lesions would later develop spasticity.

It was also recognized that some children may have diplomyelia with unilateral anomalies or hemimyelomeningocele. It is important to evaluate closely the more normal leg for loss of neurological function as a result of cord tethering from the anomalous side.

In addition, children with myelomeningocele frequently have cerebral and higher spinal cord lesions. Decreased weight of the cerebellum, cerebellar dysplasia, pyramidal tract disturbances secondary to Arnold-Chiari malformation, syringomyelia, diplomyelia, and arachnoid cysts, to mention a few, have been reported.[77] The use of magnetic resonance imaging (MRI) is recommended as a reliable test for the early detection of intraspinal pathology in myelodysplasia.[32,124]

V. PHILOSOPHY AND PRINCIPLES OF MANAGEMENT

Menelaus was direct in his statements that the aims of care in spina bifida are to establish a developmental pattern for the child which was as near normal as the level of paralysis allowed.[77] The aim of orthopedic management of the spine and lower extremities is to create a stable posture. In this regard, a minimum of flexion deformities of the hips and knees should be accepted. The center of gravity of the trunk should ideally be as close to the knee joint and anterior to the ankle joint as possible. Since the arm will be needed for the use of supportive aids in standing, the neurologic impairment of the upper extremities has special importance for standing. Sitting should be encouraged by 6 to 8 months of age and a sitting orthosis or aid may be needed at this time. At 1 to 2 years of age, standing should be encouraged and enforced. A standing frame in conjunction with appropriate lower extremity surgery should be utilized to achieve this goal (Figure 1). It is best to assume that all children who are not severely mentally retarded or who do not have gross spasticity will walk and orthopedic treatment should be directed toward this goal. Hostler points

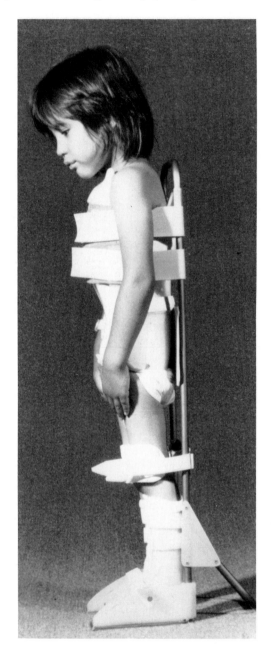

FIGURE 1. Standing frame.

out that motor actions and mental development are interrelated and that walking is not only necessary for other gross motor activities but also for socialization, language, self help, fine motor, and cognitive experiences.[45] Furthermore, prolonged sitting, especially with spinal deformity, leads to decubitus ulcers, urinary stasis, and flexion deformities. These problems can be minimized, to some degree, by developing a standing position at an early age, usually between age 1 to 2 years. In this regard special orthotic management of spinal and lower extremity deformities will be necessary in conjunction with a standing frame to achieve this goal. A parapodium can be used at age 5 to 6 years of age when the child starts school to allow sitting without orthosis removal (Figure 2).

Children with strong bilateral quadriceps function have the potential for ambulation and improved quality of life.[111] These children deserve and have the most to gain from corrective surgery of the lower extremities. Children with lower neurosegmental levels deserve aggressive treatment of the knees and feet since their potential for a high quality of life is so favorable. In contradistinction, the child with a high neurosegmental level will need more limited treatment to maintain a sitting position. A caster cart may be useful in this instance for mobility (Figure 3).

An aggressive release of muscles and tendons to create flail joints and correct fixed deformity is required. A persistence of muscle imbalance will lead to recurrent deformity. A maximum of multiple surgical corrections should be done under one anesthetic to minimize the duration of casting and therefore enhance more rapid rehabilitation. Prolonged casting is directly related to the incidence of pathologic fractures.

Orthopedic management is directed toward the goal appropriate to the neurosegmental level for the child.[52] It is useful to remember that a child's potential is reflected by the lowest active muscle innervation and this may also be complicated by spasticity. In this regard spinal cord tethering should be recognized early and treated.

Children with sacral neurosegmental levels all become community ambulators and the majority of children with thoracic neurosegmental function become sitters.[42] Stillwell and Menelaus in a related study of 50 myelomeningocele patients showed that the percentage of community ambulators within each neurosegmental group was as follows: sacral, 100%; low lumbar, 95%; high lumbar, 30%; and thoracic, 33%.[115] Their analysis revealed that mature patients, those who merely achieve household ambulation will not continue walking into adult life. Adults are either community ambulators or nonambulators.

It also must be kept in mind that all orthopedic treatment modalities must not only maximize the patient's potential and correct and minimize deformity, but also minimize the development of pressure sores. This may entail aggressive surgical correction of the deformity and appropriate total-contact orthotic treatment. Patients with a lumbar neurological deficit may be household or

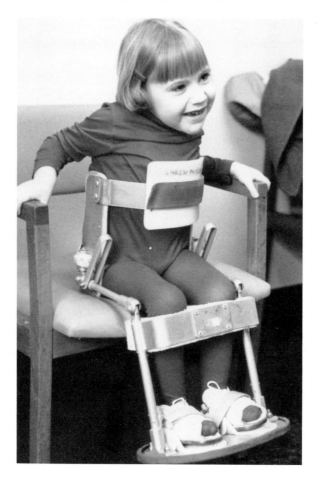

FIGURE 2. Parapodium.

community ambulators. The majority of children who have a third lumbar level deficit become functional walkers.[8] Most children become functional ambulators by age 9.[42] Treatment to make children ambulators beyond this age is not indicated.[77]

VI. THE SPINE[69]

Of all the causes of spine deformity, myelomeningocele is the most severe and most difficult to treat. In the past decade the quality of life and the life span of these children have greatly improved due to the advances in neurosurgery and urology. However, when these children become older, their spine deformity becomes an increasingly significant problem.

The treatment of these spinal deformities has advanced remarkably in the

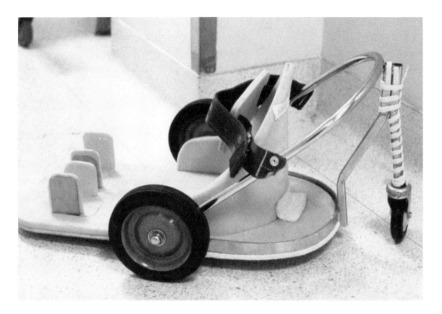

FIGURE 3. Caster cart.

last 10 to 15 years and the results of treatment have improved significantly, although several problems still exist.

Developmental or paralytic spinal deformities require orthotic support in the juvenile years and, as expected, these curves commonly progress in spite of orthotic treatment.[72] In children with higher neurosegmental deficits, skin breakdown with orthotic treatment is problematic. When paralytic scoliosis progresses beyond the limits of mechanical efficiency of bracing in the younger child, alternative treatment methods to replace long spinal fusions and resultant torso shortening have not been available. The surgical treatment of progressive scoliosis under skeletal age 10 is plagued by instrument failure due to fragile bone and skin breakdown over large and prominent instrumentation.

The surgical treatment of paralytic deformities in children over skeletal age 10 is more successful, but the problems of instrumentation failure, pseudarthrosis, and infection still remain.

Sac closure in children born with congenital lumbar kyphosis remains a problem, kyphectomy at the time of sac closure has not universally been successful, and recurrent deformity is common. Orthotic treatment is fraught with skin breakdown and progression of the kyphosis in spite of bracing is frequent. Early kyphectomy results in excessive torso shortening and unless the sacrum and pelvis are stabilized well, lumbosacral pseudarthrosis is commonplace. The surgical complications in resection of congenital lumbar kyphosis has been consistently high.

The failure of diagnosis of congenital scoliosis in the child with a paralytic curve is still a problem and can lead to a devastating outcome. The problem of the child with an unrecognized diastematomyelia, tethered cord syndrome, and progressive neurological loss is a problem that has more recently been studied,[32,77,124] and can have a permanent negative effect on functional ability ambulation potential and the development and progression of spinal deformity.[47]

A. Classification

Raycroft and Curtis reviewed 130 consecutive admissions at Newington Children's Hospital. They were able to classify two basic types of spinal deformity: the developmental or paralytic and congenital. The congenital deformities were those with anomalous vertebral development in addition to the spinal bifida. Each group was also subdivided into scoliosis, lordosis, and kyphosis.[92]

I.   Developmental (Paralytic)
    A.   Scoliosis
    B.   Kyphosis
    C.   Lordosis
    D.   Kyphoscoliosis
    E.   Lordoscoliosis
II. Congenital
    A.   Scoliosis
    B.   Kyphosis
    C.   Lordosis
III. Mixed developmental and congenital

B. Natural History

1. Developmental (Paralytic) Scoliosis

Raycroft and Curtis[93] reviewed the natural history of myelomeningocele spine deformity. In their review, 53 of the 103 patients without congenital vertebral anomalies other than spina bifida developed paralytic scoliosis, an incidence of 52%.

Of these 53 patients, 41 had scoliosis, 12 had kyphosis, and 30 had lordosis with combined deformities in many. In total, 80 of 130 patients or 62% had spine deformity, one third of the congenital types and two thirds with the paralytic type. They noted the age of curve onset in the paralytic type was 0 to 5 years = 33 patients, 6 to 10 years = 18 patients, 11 to 15 years = 2 patients, 15 to 21 years = 0 patients. Of the patients with developmental or paralytic scoliosis, 70% had uni- or bilateral hip dislocation and 83% had pelvic obliquity. They also noted a correlation between the higher level of paralysis and the greater likelihood of spine deformity. The age-related onset of spine deformity and the importance of the relationship between the level of neurologic deficit and the resultant spinal deformity was also noted by Sharrard.[98-104]

Shurleff et al.[108] analyzed 485 patients with reference to the level of neurological deficit and the age of development of "significant" scoliosis. They defined scoliosis greater than 30° to be significant. At age 1, only 3% had scoliosis. By age 10, 33% of T12 levels, 22% of the L1 to L2 levels, 18% of the L3 to L5 levels, and 3% of the S1 levels had scoliosis. By age 15, 81% of the T12 levels, 44% of the L1 to L2 levels, 23% of the L3 to L5 levels, and 9% of the S1 levels had developed significant scoliosis. At skeletal maturity it was 88, 63, 23, and 9%, respectively. Slower rates of development of scoliosis were recorded among patients with low-lumbar or asymmetrical levels of paralysis. Of these two groups, 30% were likely to acquire a scoliosis of 30° or more by adulthood.

Banta et al.[6] reviewed 268 myelodysplasia patients with at least 4 years follow-up. The incidence of scoliosis over 20° rose from 16% in the 0 to 4 age group to 50% in the 15+ age group. Those patients with defects in the thoracic and lumbar spine attained a 100% incidence of scoliosis by age 10 to 14. Those with defects in the lumbar and lumbosacral spine both attained 57 and 50% incidence, respectively, of scoliosis by the age of 15. The incidence of scoliosis increased in each succeedingly older age group, with the most dramatic increases noted in the less ambulatory or higher level paralysis patients.

Hall and Martin[38] reviewed 130 patients with myelomeningocele at skeletal maturity. They observed that 101 or 78% had clinical spine deformity.

Mackel and Lindseth[65] in their review of 82 patients with myelomeningocele followed for 10 years found that the overall incidence of scoliosis was 66%, including both developmental and congenital curves. The incidence of scoliosis was highest in the patients with thoracic-level paraplegia (100%) and gradually decreased to 70% with L4 paraplegia. All curves appeared within the first decade and progressed relentlessly.

According to Moe et al.,[79] one can expect a 100% incidence of spinal deformity at T12 level paraplegia or above, 90% at L1, 80% at L2, 70% at L3, 60% at L4, 25% at L5, and 5% at S1. Development curves will gradually develop before age 10, will be associated with a rapid increase during the adolescent growth spurt, and then progress until skeletal maturity or longer. They are frequently associated with pelvic obliquity which commonly becomes fixed and may result in loss of sitting stability. Developmental scoliosis is usually associated with lordosis and hip flexion contractures are commonplace.

Piggott[91] noted that in his series of 191 children with myelomeningocele, 82.5% had scoliosis, 17.5% had kyphosis, 12.5% had lordosis, and 10% had no deformity. The most significant finding in his study was that by age 10, 90% of children had some degree of deformity. It was also apparent that the frequency of deformity was related to neurologic deficit: 83% of children with neurologic deficit above T12 had scoliosis and 67% with neurologic deficit between L1 and the sacrum had scoliosis. In addition, the causes of scoliosis were evident. Thirty-eight percent were due to congenital causes, 62% were due to paralysis, 15% were due to asymmetric neural arch and associated muscle attachment, and 12% were "idiopathic" curves.

2. Developmental (Paralytic) Kyphosis

Kyphosis of greater than 35° in the lumbar spine or greater than 65° for the whole spine was considered significant according to Raycroft and Curtis.[93] At age 2, 27% of patients with T12 level had developed significant kyphosis. By age 10, 35% of T12 level, 0% of the L1 to L2 levels, 2% of the L3 to L5 levels, and 9% of the S1 levels had developed kyphosis. At skeletal maturity 62, 12, 2, and 9%, respectively, were noted to have "significant" kyphosis. Their incidence of developmental kyphosis was 12% in agreement with Hoppenfeld.[44]

3. Developmental (Paralytic) Lordosis

Lordosis was more prevalent in the higher level cases and increased with age irrespective of motor levels. Of those patients with T12 or higher deficits, 58% had lordosis by age 4 and 100% by age 15. Of those with L3 to L4 lesions, 60% had lordosis by age 4 and 80% by age 15. Of those with S1 lesions, 20% had lordosis by age 4 and 40% by age 15.[93]

4. Congenital Scoliosis

The natural history of congenital scoliosis other than spina bifida is similar to congenital scoliosis without spina bifida.[86,128] Many patients with myelomeningocele have a mixture of congenital and paralytic (developmental) spine deformity. In contradistinction to the developmental curvatures that are usually flexible until late, the congenital curve is usually rigid and progresses early in childhood.

According to Raycroft and Curtis,[93] all of the patients at Newington Children's Hospital who had congenital defects of the vertebral bodies developed congenital spine deformity. In addition, the congenital curvatures usually had some spinal deformity at birth in contradistinction to the paralytic type.

5. Congenital Kyphosis

Congenital kyphosis in myelodysplasia is evident in 8 to 15% of patients.[34,44,108] It is usually located in the lumbar spine and frequently measures 80 to 90° at birth.[27,103] These children usually have a T12 level paraplegia and skin closures at birth may be difficult. The kyphosis is rigid,[44] and usually progresses during infancy, commonly reaching 120° by age 3.[79] The average rate of progression is 8°/year.[5] Respiratory compromise may be associated with progression of this deformity due to incompetence of the respiratory muscles and crowding of the abdominal contents and upward pressure on the diaphragm.[59]

Hoppenfeld[44] described the pathologic anatomy of the spine in children with congenital lumbar kyphosis. In his dissections of necropsy material from newborn infants, he noted that in the kyphotic spine, the pedicles were widely spaced in the area of the deformity and protruded posterolaterally. The lumbar facets were rotated anterolaterally and were in the coronal plane instead of the normal sagittal plane. The paraspinal muscles were laterally displaced and found next to the pedicles. The pelvis was rotated forward and the plane of the lower limbs were at right angles to that of the trunk, projecting an appearance of severe hip flexion contractures.

Drennan also performed anatomic dissections in 12 cases of congenital kyphosis. He noted that the erector spinae and quadratus lumborum muscles, instead of being posterior to the spine, were anterolateral and thus mechanically functioned as spinal flexors. In addition, the psoas was found to be far anterior to the apex of the kyphosis, thus having the capability of aggravating the kyphosis.[27]

C. Nonoperative Treatment
1. Developmental Scoliosis

Although it has been well accepted that nonoperative orthotic treatment plays a valuable and specific role in the overall treatment program in these patients, very little information has been published concerning results of this treatment. At present, orthotic treatment is primarily directed toward the developmental or paralytic curvature. The patients with paralytic scoliosis usually develop long "C-shaped" curvatures frequently associated with pelvic obliquity at a relatively young age (Figure 4). The purpose of bracing is to control curve progression and maintain trunk balance until the optimum age for fusion. Long spinal fusions before skeletal age 10 will result in a great loss of trunk height due to stunting of growth. It is better to brace the curve for several years until the onset of the adolescent growth spurt and then proceed with the desired spinal fusion. The ideal age for the definitive spinal fusion is around age 10 to 11 in girls and age 12 to 13 in boys (Figure 5). In general, children with myelomeningocele mature earlier than normal children as a consequence earlier spine fusion is not as inappropriate as it may appear from a chronological standpoint. If curve progression continues in spite of bracing, subcutaneous Moe instrumentation can be performed without fusion. This instrumentation, in conjunction with bracing, frequently can control curve progression until the optimum time for fusion.[80] Spinal bracing usually does not avoid the need for fusion but will delay the timing of the arthrodesis.

Patients with developmental deformity with pure scoliosis, kyphoscoliosis, or lordoscoliosis are the best candidates for brace treatment. The indications for treatment are deformities of 20° or more as noted on upright sitting films.[79] All progressive deformities should be braced before fixed deformity develops. The child may need several brace changes during growth.

Although absence of skin sensation is not a contraindication, there are two contraindications to orthotic treatment. First, if the child is obese and a desired fit cannot be achieved, then it is futile to continue. Second, if the parent cannot

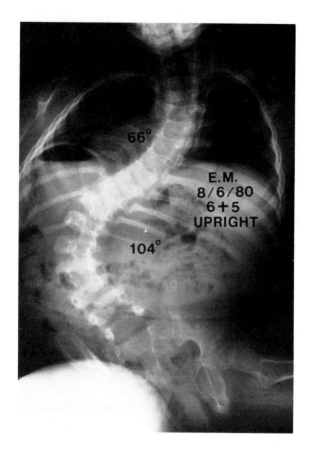

FIGURE 4. E.M. with lumbar L2-3 neurosegmental level developed a severe paralytic scoliosis by age 6+5.

provide the care needed in the time-consuming program, then bracing is contraindicated.[12]

Orthotic treatment should be stopped under three circumstances:

1. If curve progression occurs in spite of adequate bracing and subcutaneous instrumentation does not seem feasible, then spinal fusion should be planned.
2. If the patient cannot tolerate continued skin pressure, then it is inadvisable to continue with orthotic treatment.
3. If the patient has reached skeletal age 10 to 12, then spinal fusion should not be delayed since adequate spinal growth has been attained by this age.

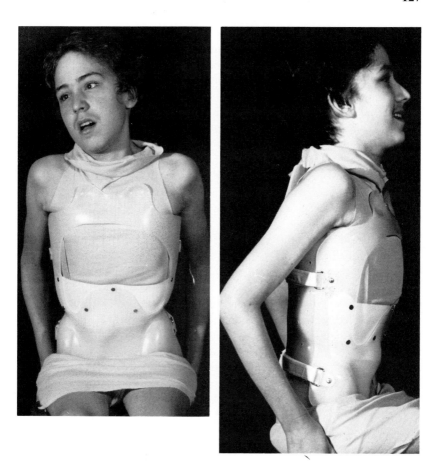

A   B

FIGURE 5. (A) Bivalved body jacket, front view. (B) Bivalved body jacket, back view.

2. Congenital Scoliosis

Congenital curvatures are frequently rigid and respond poorly to orthotic treatment. However, in the patient with mixed deformities (i.e., congenital and paralytic), the paralytic curve can successfully be braced, but the congenital or anomalous area should be closely watched. If progression occurs in the anomalous area of the spine, a selective arthrodesis should be performed, thus converting the curve to a purely paralytic pattern. Orthotic treatment in this situation should be continued.

3. Kyphosis

In developmental kyphosis bracing, though it is more difficult, it can be useful and long radius deformities are more responsive than short radius curvatures. In contradistinction, congenital kyphosis is usually unresponsive to brace treatment and is not recommended.

The underarm brace has been the most widely used brace in children with myelomeningocele. In general, although the modified Milwaukee brace[12] may be useful in the orthotic treatment of thoracic curves, the underarm bivalved body jacket is recommended for most paralytic curves. The design concept that the author finds useful is the interlocking bivalved body jacket with Velcro straps (Figure 6). It is designed to offer ease of application and removal.[128] Other techniques have been advocated; Drennan has advocated the use of gravity in conjunction with underarm bracing by suspending the patient and the brace in a wheelchair using special brackets.[26]

D. Operative Treatment
1. Preoperative Evaluation

A thorough evaluation of each child undergoing surgical treatment of their spine deformity is imperative. An analysis of the three-dimensional deformity and the functional problems that it creates, the quality of the skin over the back and abdomen, the extent of the laminal defect, the presence and degree of hip flexion contractures, and pelvic obliquity should be done.

In addition to a general medical evaluation it is essential that any hydrocephalus is stationary and any cerebral shunts are functional. Perhaps more importantly, a complete evaluation of the urologic system is a prerequisite before any surgical procedure on the spine is undertaken. Any obstructive uropathy should be solved and any active urinary infection should be thoroughly treated.

It is important that the various spine curvatures be evaluated completely before embarking upon a surgical program and certain roentgenograms are useful:

1.   Sitting anteroposterior and lateral spine films for general curve and degree of pelvic obliquity measurement
2.   Supine traction anteroposterior films to determine the degree of scoliosis flexibility
3.   Supine hyperextension lateral films to determine the degree of kyphosis correction
4.   A supine lateral film of the lumbosacral spine in the knee-chest position to evaluate the degree of fixed lumbar lordosis

Every child should be assessed relative to their ambulatory capacity, presence and degree of hip flexion contractures, and muscle strength grading of the lower extremities prior to surgery. Staged releases of hip flexion contractures may be necessary before correction of severe lumbar lordosis in some children or their ambulatory potential may be compromised.

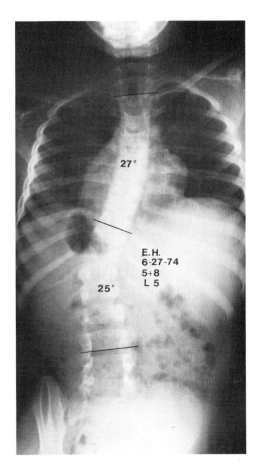

A

FIGURE 6. (A) E.H. (L5 neurosegmental level) at age 5+8 had developed a 27° right thoracic and a 25° left thoracolumbar paralytic scoliosis. (B) E.H. at age 9+8, the thoracolumbar scoliosis had progressed to 41° during orthotic treatment. (C) E.H. at age 10+10, her curve had progressed to 83° out of the brace. (D) E.H. 1 year after staged instrumentation and fusion.

2. General Principles

Several general principles are applicable in the surgical treatment of these spinal deformities: (1) preservation of respiratory function, (2) maintenance of sitting stability, (3) a level pelvis, and (4) maximum torso length with minimal bony prominences.

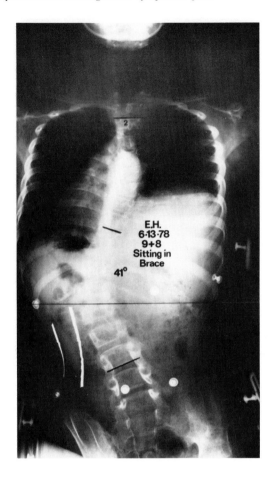

FIGURE 6B.

The selection of the fusion area is critical. The most common error usually has been the selection of an inadequate fusion area. The same principles with all neuromuscular curves apply. Fusion to the sacrum is necessary in most collapsing and paralytic curves. The upper proximal extent of the fusion should be one or two vertebra above the uppermost vertebra of the paralytic curve as measured on the upright film. This applies to both anterior and posterior fusions for scoliosis, kyphosis, lordosis, or a combination thereof.[79]

In patients with congenital spine deformity, the entire extent of the curve must be fused. In patients with mixed congenital and paralytic curves, the longer fusion area dictated by the paralytic curve should apply.

In congenital lumbar kyphosis the entire length of the deformity must be

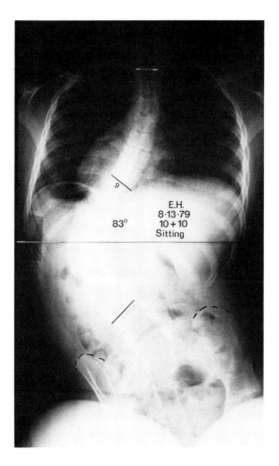

FIGURE 6C.

fused. The proximal extent should be at least two vertebra above the proximal extent of the kyphosis and the distal extent of the fusion should include the sacrum. In general, anything short of this will be associated with progression of the kyphotic deformity.

3. Operative Technique

Each patient is unique and the operative techniques will have to be tailored individually. It has been well established that the best results in treating paralytic curvatures have been achieved when combined anterior and posterior fusions and instrumentation is employed.[70–72,75] In children older than age 10 with lumbar scoliosis and lordosis, staged anterior fusion to the sacrum utilizing Zielke or Dwyer instrumentation to L5 or S1 and posterior fusion and Harrington or Cotrel Dubousset instrumentation to the sacrum should be done (Figure 5). Segmental spinal instrumentation (SSI) has been advocated in myelomeningocele spine deformity[3,4,64,118] (Figure 7). Although segmental

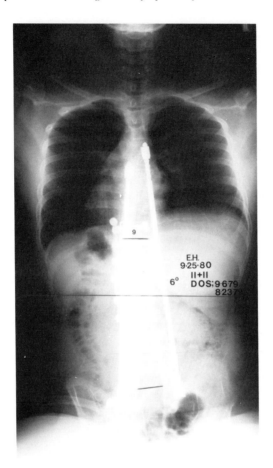

FIGURE 6D.

posterior instrumentation system is biomechanically stronger than the standard Harrington system, long-term results are incomplete.

It is extremely helpful to avoid the scarred, potentially infected midline area from previous sac resection by using a "Y" incision.[70] The bifurcation should begin at the upper extent of the laminal defect and each arm should then parallel the bony everted laminal area to the sacrum. The skin incision can utilize the "Y" technique as well if the midline skin is of poor quality, but if the midline skin is good a midline skin incision is preferable.

It is recommended that all rod implants be contoured to the residual lordosis and kyphosis. An acute lordotic bend of the distal end of the Harrington distraction rod is imperative for proper seating and fixation of the sacral hook.

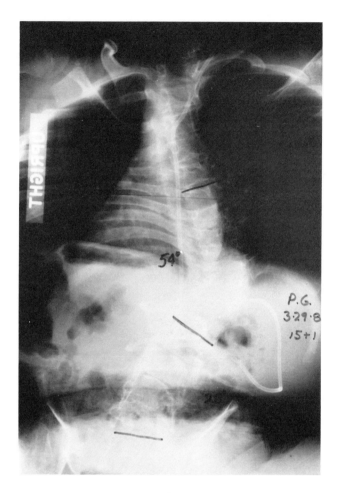

A

FIGURE 7. (A) P.G. (neurosegmental level T12) had developed a 54° right thoracic scoliosis. (B) P.G. after Cotrel-Dubousset segmental instrumentation.

The square-ended Harrington rod should be used in all patients to prevent rod rotation. Segmental wiring of the Harrington rods can be performed including as many vertebral levels as technically feasible.

Anterior Dwyer or Zielke instrumentation should extend to S1 if possible but certainly L4 or L5 should be instrumented (Figure 5). However, a screw head must not protrude underneath the common iliac artery or vein. If the

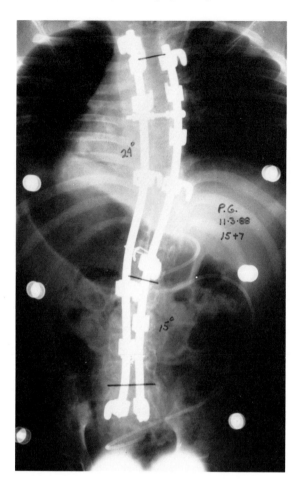

FIGURE 7B.

anterior instrumentation must stop short of S1, then, if technically possible, the anterior fusion should extend to the sacrum since the lumbosacral area is the most common location for pseudarthrosis.

The Dwyer and Zielke instruments are effective in correcting lordosis and rotational kyphosis but not sagittal nonrotational kyphosis. Traction prior to surgery has not been found helpful.

Autogenous bone graft should be used from both iliac crests. In addition, abundant bank bone should be used. Osebold et al.[86] has shown that the use of bank bone has not adversely affected the fusion rate. In his series of 40 patients, those patients who received combined autogenous and bank bone graft had fewer pseudarthroses than those patients who received autogenous bone alone.

E. Postoperative Management

The standard postoperative brace is a bivalved polypropylene body jacket made from a plaster model of the patient taken on a Risser frame after surgical correction (Figure 6). The hips are not immobilized. The patient returns to upright activities as soon as the brace fits well. The brace is worn 24 h/d but can be removed frequently with the patient in the supine position for skin care. The brace is worn until the fusion is solid — usually 6 to 12 months.

1. Congenital Scoliosis

Patients with congenital scoliosis and myelomeningocele usually require a fusion at a younger age than those who have developmental curves. Those patients who have a unilateral unsegmented bar should have an *in situ* fusion as soon as the diagnosis is recognized. If the bar is in the laminal defect area, an osteotomy of the bar can be performed in conjunction with staged anterior and posterior fusion and instrumentation. In performing the osteotomy, care should be taken, however, to avoid the dural sac.

In those patients who have a lumbar scoliosis with pelvic obliquity and one or two hemivertebrae in the lumbar curve, a staged anterior fusion without hemivertebra excision followed by bilateral transverse process fusion as a second stage can be done without instrumentation in the younger child when progression of the scoliosis is evident.

Hemivertebra excision is not recommended except in severe and rigid lumbar curves where the pelvic obliquity cannot be corrected by any other means. In this situation, a two-stage hemivertebra excision should be done but compression instrumentation should be used on the convex side to close the wedge or a recurrence of the deformity will occur. If inadequate bone stock for hook purchase is a problem, then end-fusions can be performed as advocated by Marchetti[68] 4 months before the excision and instrumentation is done. This has been particularly useful in patients with hemimyelomeningocele (Figure 8).

An alternative method of correcting fixed pelvic obliquity was described by Lindseth.[57] He advocated bilateral pelvic osteotomies with simultaneous opening and closing wedges. This technique was successful in nine patients with 2 to 7 year follow-up.

Occasionally some patients may have two areas of anomalies, one in the thoracic area and another in the lumbar spine associated with spina bifida. These areas may be fused separately and the intervening areas of the spine treated orthotically. Later, when adequate spine growth has occurred, a longer fusion incorporating these areas may be necessary.

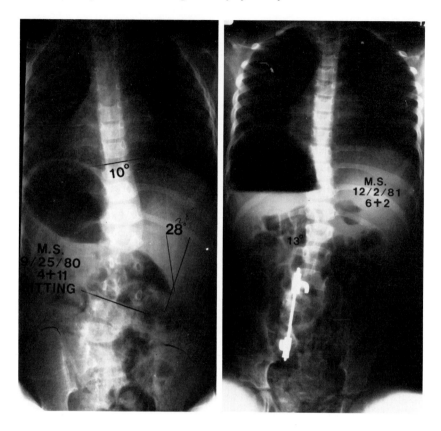

A   B

FIGURE 8. (A) M.S. (neurosegmental level L4) at age 4+11 had developed a progressive 28°
right thoracolumbar scoliosis as a result of a lumbrosacral hemivertebra. (B) M.S. after hemivertebra excision and compression instrumentation at age 6+2.

2. Congenital Lumbar Kyphosis

Sharrard pioneered resection of the kyphosis, particularly in the newborn,
in order to gain skin closure.[104] Lindseth and Stelzer[59] in 1979 advocated
resection of the lordotic component of the deformity with wire fixation and
limited fusion at the resected apex at age 3 to 4 years. Unfortunately, 9 of 12
patients had progression of their deformity within the first year after surgery.
Long-term studies, however, have not been reported.

Hall and Poitra[39] stated, "Correction can be accomplished only by excision
of the bony elements of the kyphosis, but maintenance of correction can be
obtained only by solid interbody and posterior fusion of the entire length of the
deformity." It has been the experience of this author that their observation has
held true. They reported six cases treated by sac excision, kyphectomy, and
compression rod fixation at age 3 to 8 years.

In the child under age 3 with a large deformity that is progressing, an anterior strut graft fusion will stabilize the kyphosis. Further resection of the kyphotic deformity can be done at an older age.

In the child over 5 years of age, a formal resection of the kyphosis as described by Hall and Poitra[39] is recommended. The midline skin is elliptically excised, the incisions paralleling the lateral bony ridges. The proximal and distal limbs of the excision are in the midline. The entire spinal cord and sac are removed. This is only done in the child with complete flaccid paraplegia of T12 or higher. The entire spinal canal is cleaned of soft tissue distally to the lowest level of the sacrum. The proximal portion of the sac is transected at the level of the normal lamina. The dura is closed with a pursestring ligature. The spinal cord is never tied off. Acute hydrocephalus has been reported due to closure of the central canal of the spinal cord.[127] Bleeding, as a result of this resection, can be excessive and is usually controlled by cautery and bone wax. The dissection is then carried out subperiosteally around the anterior vertebral bodies. The lordotic portion of the spine is osteomized and then resected including vertebral bodies, pedicles, and everted laminae. The remaining lumbar discs are resected. Compression instrumentation is usually sufficient for smaller children[39] (Figure 9). In older children, the author advocates supplementing the compression instrumentation, which functions by creating interfragmentary fixation, with distraction rods or the use of segmental instrumentation[41,76] (Figure 10). A posterior spinal fusion is then performed. Two weeks later, an anterior strut graft or inlay fusion is performed. About 5 to 7 d after the second stage fusion, a model for a bivalved body jacket is taken and when fitted, the patient may resume an upright posture. The brace is worn until the fusion is solid, usually 6 to 9 months.

VII. RESULTS AND COMPLICATIONS

Sriram et al. in 1972[117] reported on their experience with the surgical management of these deformities from only a posterior spinal approach. In their series, they reported a pseudarthrosis rate of 44% and a wound infection rate of 22%.

Hull et al.,[48] in 1974 evaluated results in 33 patients surgically treated with follow-up of more than 1 year. Their overall infection rate was 67%. There were three deaths and five patients developed cast sores.

Osebold et al.[86] reviewed the historical evolution of the surgical treatment of paralytic curves in Minneapolis-St. Paul. They found that the best results were achieved when combined anterior and posterior instrumentation and arthrodesis was utilized. With this combined approach, the pseudarthrosis rate was 23% and the wound infection rate was 8%.

Mayfield in 1981[70] reported on 19 patients with paralytic scoliosis treated surgically utilizing staged anterior and posterior fusion with Dwyer or Zielke and posterior Harrington instrumentation as well as autogenous and bank bone

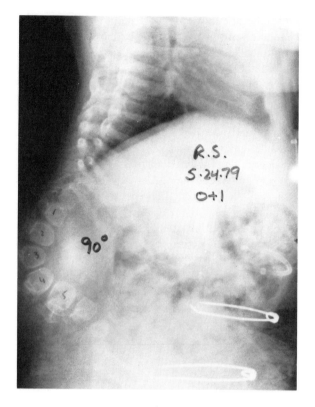

A

FIGURE 9. (A) R.S. (neurosegmental level T12) at age 1 month had a 90° congenital lumbar kyphosis. (B) R.S. at age 4+0. The kyphosis had progressed to 134°. (C) R.S. at age 4+4. The kyphosis had been stabilized with an anterior vascularized rib graft. (D) R.S. at age 7+9, 2 years after kyphectomy and posterior cable-hook instrumentation.

graft. The pseudarthrosis rate was 20%. All patients were evaluated preoperatively for urinary infection and those patients with urinary infections were treated with intravenous antibiotics for 7 to 10 d prior to surgery. With this protocol, no postoperative wound infections were noted.

In general, the results of surgery in paralytic scoliosis in myelomeningocele are significantly better combined anterior and posterior fusions and rigid anterior and posterior instrumentation were utilized.[70,72,75] These surgical techniques combined with the use of bank and autogenous bone graft bone decreased the pseudarthrosis rate significantly. The results using more rigid segmental spinal instrumentation (SSI) have not yet been reported.

Long-term results in the surgical treatment of congenital lumbar kyphosis are few. Lindseth and Stelzer in 1979[59] reported on their experience with

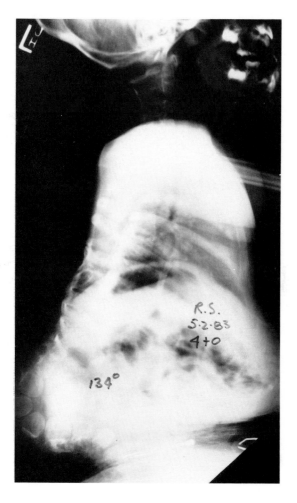

FIGURE 9B.

vertebral excision in 23 patients. They advocated resection of the lordotic component of the deformity with fixation of the resected spine with wire or mersilene tape. Of 12 patients treated in this fashion, 9 had progression of their deformity 1 year postoperatively and 4 had further progression of the kyphosis 4 years postoperatively. All 12 patients, however, gained an average of 1.5 cm in height due to growth. Complications included urinary tract infections, decubitus ulcer in one patient, and wound infections in 7 out of 23 patients (30%).

McMaster reported on 10 patients followed for 7 years, 4 months after kyphectomy. They concluded that the best results were with the use of long rigid instrumentation and fusions. Complications were high.[76] Dunn, in 1983,[29] reviewed his experience in the surgical treatment of 15 patients with lumbar

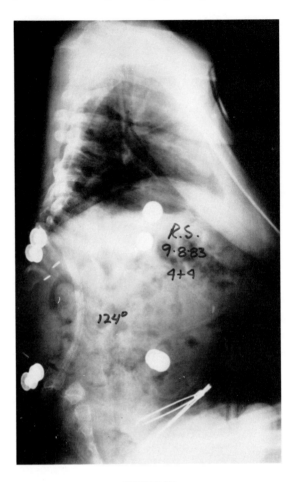

FIGURE 9C.

kyphosis since 1971. Complications included wound infection, acute hydro-cephalus, excessive torso shortening, nonunion, and skin breakdown over the prominent instrumentation. In his experience, segmental spinal instrumenta-tion is an improvement due to the improved fixation but no long-term studies are available.

Mayfield and King in 1983[71] reported on the use of flexible cable-hook compression system for instrumentation in conjunction with resection of the lordotic component of the spine deformity, spinal cord excision, and combined anterior and posterior arthrodeses. The mean kyphosis preoperatively was 127° and the mean kyphosis correction was 113°. Of the seven patients in this small series, one was lost to follow-up and the remaining six had a solid fusion at follow-up. Although the results were good in this series, the follow-up was

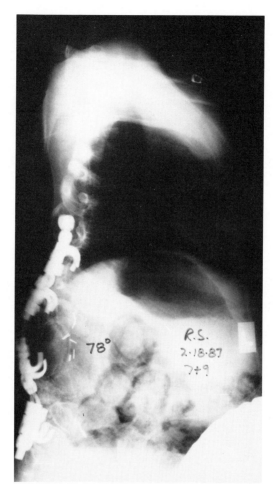

FIGURE 9D.

short (mean 18 months). Although significant correction and maintenance of correction of the kyphotic deformity was achieved in this series, it was necessary to fuse most of the lumbar spine, a distinct disadvantage in the child under age 5. Complications included fluid overload due to overtransfusion and skin breakdown over prominent instrumentation. There were no wound infections.

Heydermann reported in 1988 on the results of kyphectomy with long posterior segmental Luque instrumentation. With follow-up of 6 to 57 months, only one patient lost correction. A single-stage posterior fusion and instrumentation were recommended.[41]

In summary, a complete solution to the problem of lumbar kyphosis has not yet been found. Inadequate correction and fixation in hopes of preserving

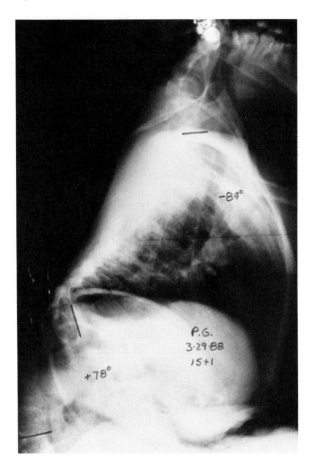

A

FIGURE 10.   (A) P.G. at age 15+1 (Neurosegmental level T12) had 78° congenital lumbar kyphosis. (B) P.G. 6 months after staged kyphectomy and segmental Cotrel-Dubousset instrumentation.

growth usually leads to failure. Aggressive correction with rigid instrumentation and fusion of the entire deformity leads to permanent correction in older children but leads to significant torso shortening in the young child.

VIII. HEMIMYELOMENINGOCELE

Hemimyelodysplasia is an unusual spectrum of congenital anomalies of the spine, sacrum, and pelvis associated with one normal leg and the other totally or near totally paralyzed.[66] The roentgenograms show anomalous vertebral development in addition to the spina bifida. Both failures of vertebral formation and segmentation are noted. Sacral hypoplasia is common. Interpedicular

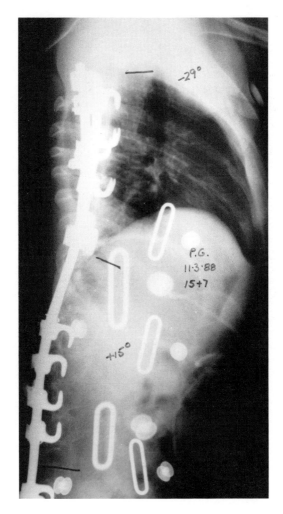

FIGURE 10B.

widening is commonplace and associated diastematomyelia may be present.[66] Spinal cord tethering may be seen and 60% have renal anomalies.[66]

The orthopedic management is complex and is directed toward the spinal deformity and leg length discrepancy. Congenital or paralytic foot and leg problems such as knee contractures or clubfeet may require prompt, ongoing treatment.

The most common problem is a progressive lumbar scoliosis due to asymmetric growth of anomalous vertebrae. These anomalies are usually located at lumbosacral junction and the resultant deformity is pelvic obliquity with lateral torso deviation (Figure 11).

The leg length discrepancy is due to neurologic deficit and pelvic obliquity.

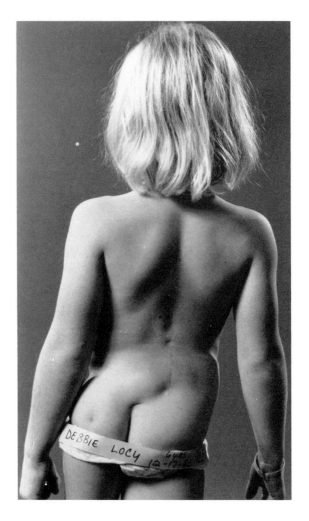

A

FIGURE 11. (A) D.L. clinical appearance at age 6. Hemimyelomeningocele. (B) D.L. Note hypoplastic left leg. (C) D.L. Radiographic appearance of hemimyelomeningocele. Note lumbosacral bar and hemivertebrae and subluxed left hip. (D) D.L. after staged wedge resection and fusion.

The discrepancy may be severe and may require equalization procedures, including leg lengthening.

The treatment of the spinal deformity necessitates wedge resection at the lumbosacral area in order to achieve adequate compensation. Adequate correction requires sufficient wedge resection anteriorly and posteriorly as well as good internal fixation (Figure 11).

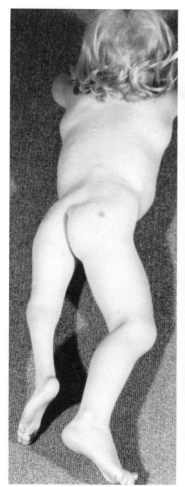

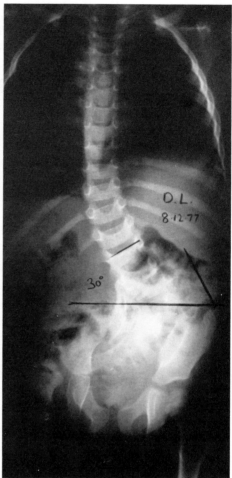

FIGURE 11B.   FIGURE 11C.

IX. THE HIP

Menelaus has aptly stated that there are three aims of treatment of the hip deformity and disability: (1) to treat hip deformity and dislocation only in those children who will thrive and benefit significantly from such treatment, (2) to perform only a single operation on each hip, and (3) to minimize the duration of postoperative immobilization.[77,78]

The primary cause of hip abnormalities in myelomeningocele is muscle imbalance. This muscle imbalance produces abnormal forces across the hip joint leading to growth alterations of the proximal femur and acetabulum. Mechanically these secondary bony deformities coupled with muscle imbalance may lead to subluxation or dislocation. The acetabulum becomes increas-

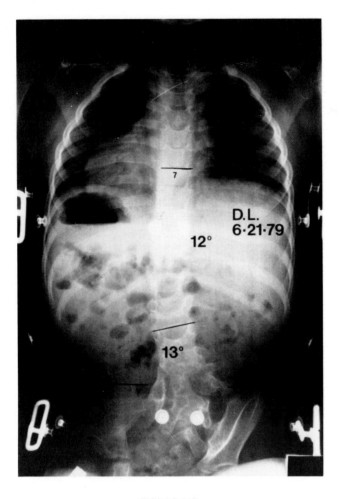

FIGURE 11D.

ingly deficient and fetal coxa valga persists due to muscle imbalance and limited weight bearing.

A. Principles of Treatment

Long-term follow-up studies indicate that reduction of the hips is not a prerequisite for ambulation[35,105] (Figure 12). A level pelvis and a good range of hip motion are more important for function than hip reduction.[35] The most important variable affecting ambulation is the level of paralysis and in the child with L3 and L4 neurosegmental function musculoskeletal and hip deformity (not dislocation) more directly related to ambulation.[2] It has been shown that the presence of the femoral head in the acetabulum does not improve range of hip motion or ability to walk nor does it reduce the amount of bracing required

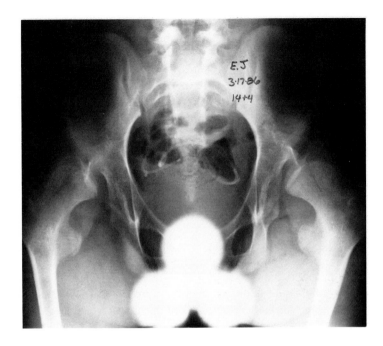

FIGURE 12. E.J., L4 neurosegmental level. At age 14+4 patient is a community ambulator with bilateral hip dislocations.

or decrease pain and a gluteus medius lurch persisted irrespective of the presence of hip reduction or muscle transfers.[35]

Major hip surgery is only appropriate for those children who have strong quadriceps function bilaterally and therefore have the potential for household or community ambulation.[77,78] The aim of treatment is to provide hips that can assume a position of full extension and will not become deformed. Therefore, in high lumbar lesions, surgery should be restricted to muscle and contracture releases and in low lumbar lesion more extensive hip surgery is justified.

Iliopsoas transplantation and reduction of hip dislocation should be reserved for children who will have a good quality of life, who have strong quadriceps strength, and will ambulate with below-the-knee braces.[77,125] In iliopsoas transplantation, 67% poor results in upper lumbar lesions and 17% poor results in lower lumbar lesions have been reported.[87] Furthermore, the actual value of iliopsoas transfers is in question because of the variability of results. This presently is an unanswered question.

B. Hip Splinting

The use of a hip splint from birth to age 1 or 2 years to stimulate acetabular development and promote hip stability has been advocated.[74,97] Although the efficiency of splinting has not been verified in long-term studies, it is the author's experience that some benefit can be derived by minimizing acetabular dysplasia which may be useful if surgical treatment is required later. A COH abduction flexion splint or Pavlik Harness have been useful in this regard.

Most of the hip disorders in spina bifida can be treated by one or a combination of the following procedures:[77,97]

1. Radical hip release to correct flexion, abduction, and lateral rotation deformity after age $2^1/_2$ years[107]
2. Division of adductors and iliopsoas to prevent recurrent deformity
3. Anterior hip release to correct flexion deformity
4. Adductor release and iliopsoas or external oblique transfer
5. Acetabuloplasty
6. Proximal femoral osteotomy

C. Soft Tissue Procedures

Many children with myelomeningocele and thoracic or high lumbar lesions lie with their legs in a position of abduction, flexion, and external rotation. If the range of internal rotation is unaltered by flexion of the hip, then the psoas is not responsible for the deformity. In order to prevent abduction and external rotation contractures from developing, the legs should be held together with a sleeve. Once an abduction external rotation contracture has developed, then a radical hip release is necessary. This may require a combination of iliopsoas release, abductor and iliotibial band and tensor fascia lateral release, and external rotator release. This may need to be combined with posterior capsule release and anterior capsule reefing. Postoperatively, the child is maintained in traction with the legs in adduction and extension in conjunction with physiotherapy.

Division of the iliopsoas and adductors is indicated when flexion and adduction deformities are a problem.[125] A section of psoas tendon can be excised to prevent recurrence. Postoperatively the child is held in abduction casts for 6 weeks.

Tendon transfers fall into two categories: iliopsoas transfer and external oblique transfer. Both of these procedures are reserved for children with excellent walking potential, who have muscle imbalance at the hip, and who have strong quadriceps function bilaterally. The iliopsoas tendon may be transferred posterior (Sharrard) or laterally (Mustard). The external oblique transfer is a lateral transfer. Other pathologic conditions about the hip should be corrected at the same time as the transfer with concomitant procedures: (1) adductor release to correct adduction contracture, (2) anterior capsular plication if subluxation or dislocation is present, (3) acetabuloplasty to correct acetabular dysplasia, and (4) proximal femoral varus osteotomy to correct persistent valgus or rotational deformity.

Historically, the lateral iliopsoas transfer as described by Mustard has not been effective in preventing subluxation or dislocation.[17,97] The posterior iliopsoas transfer was described by Sharrard in 1959.[99] The main purpose of the transfer was to remove the deformity force of the iliopsoas and transfer it to the posterior greater trochanter and convert it to an active extensor and abductor. There is a wide variation of reported results from the posterolateral iliopsoas transfer from good results[11,78,87,95,130] to poor results.[50,92] This may be the result of other abnormalities about the hip that may or may not have been corrected at the time of the transfer. Shafer and Dias[97] emphasize several factors:

1. Either an adductor myotomy or adductor transfer is always indicated.
2. If the hip is dislocated, capsular plication is necessary.
3. If the acetabular index is over 25°, acetabuloplasty should be done.
4. If more than 25° of abduction and internal rotation are necessary to keep the hip stable, a varus osteotomy should be done.
5. Care should be used not to damage the innervation to the sartorius in exposure.
6. At closure the sartorius and rectus should be reattached to the ilium.

Patient selection in posterolateral iliopsoas transfer is important.[11,125] Bunch reported in his series of 32 children that all had L4 neurosegmental function and 21 (66%) had active function with good results. In his series more commonly good results were seen when a varus osteotomy was done as well.[11]

The external oblique transfer was described by Lowman.[63] Thomas modified the transfer so that all of the muscle was used.[120] Ynque and Lindseth reported improved results in 57% of children with external oblique transfer. It has several advantages over the iliopsoas transfer: (1) it does not weaken the hip when transferred, (2) muscle power is added to the hip, (3) it is a synergistic transfer instead of an antagonistic transfer.[97,120]

D. Bony Procedures

Progressive coxa valga and increased femoral anteversion is common in paralytic hip dislocation in spina bifida. Varus derotation osteotomy has been advocated to correct proximal femoral deformity as a result of muscle imbalance in myelomeningocele[51] (Figure 13). This has been effective, and to avoid a recurrent angle of 90°, varus has been recommended as well as bilateral varus derotation osteotomies to avoid unilateral femoral head uncovering on the opposite hip.[46] Dias reported 24 out of 28 hips stable after varus derotation osteotomies.[19,97] The varus derotation osteotomy frequently is done with other procedures to correct adaptive bony changes (pelvic osteotomy), release contractures (adductor and iliopsoas release), or with muscle transfers (iliopsoas or external oblique transfers). It should be kept in mind that it is preferable to correct any pelvic obliquity before surgical correction of hip subluxation or dislocation or failure may ensue.

Pelvic osteotomy should be considered when acetabular dysplasia is present. The Pemberton osteotomy[90] is a stable osteotomy and is useful when the acetabulum is broad and shallow. The Chiari osteotomy[16] is useful when the

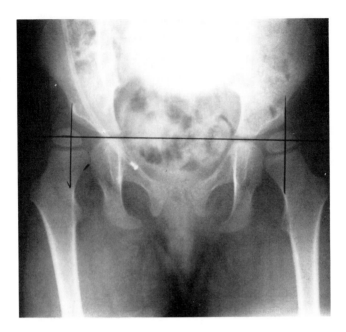

A

FIGURE 13. (A) L4 Neurosegmental function. Bilateral hip subluxation.
(B) Bilateral varus derotation osteotomies and external oblique transfers.

femoral head is partially dislocated and reduction is not planned and when the acetabulum is very small and deficient (Figure 14). The Steele osteotomy[115] has been employed when the acetabulum is severely maldirected. The Salter osteotomy[96] and Steele osteotomies are generally not used in myelodysplasia since acetabular deficiency is present rather than maldirection.

Acetabuloplasty is combined with one or more of the following: adductor or iliopsoas release, iliopsoas transfer, varus derotation osteotomy, or open reduction and capsular plication.

Pelvic obliquity can adversely effect hip subluxation or dislocation. In addition, unequal pressure distribution on the ischium can cause skin breakdown.[28] Pelvic obliquity may be infra- or suprapelvic. Suprapelvic causes are primarily due to scoliosis and should be addressed with timely orthotic treatment in conjunction with appropriate surgical correction and fusion. Infrapelvic causes should be addressed during all ages of treatment in hopes of preventing fixed deformity. When a fixed pelvic obliquity is present and the scoliosis and infrapelvic causes have been corrected, bilateral corrective pelvic osteotomies have been described to level the pelvis.[60,85] Lindseth[57] has reported good results with this procedure.

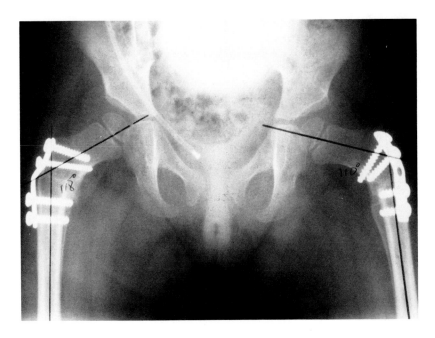

FIGURE 13B.

X. THE KNEE

The presence of strong quadriceps determines the effectiveness of ambulation. It is often difficult to determine if the quadriceps are strong enough to allow only below-the-knee orthosis until the child is older. Therefore, Menelaus suggests delaying decisions concerning surgical treatment of the hip until this decision can be made.[77]

Flexion contractures are the most common problem and suggest weak quadriceps with or without hamstring spasm. Reflex hamstring spasm is most frequently seen in children with thoracolumbar lesions. Parsch and Manner[88] noted in their series of patients that flexion or valgus knee deformities were present in 50% of thoracolumbar lesions, 20% of lumbar lesions, and 15% of sacral lesions. When strong hamstrings seem to be problematic, transfer of their insertion to the distal femur is recommended.[31] In their series, Abraham et al. found that the lowest incidence of recurrence was noted in children who had hamstring transfers to the patella.[1] In more rigid fixed flexion deformities, radical posterior capsular knee and hamstring release may be necessary. In the older child, supracondylar osteotomy of the femur may be necessary but should be a last resort.

Hyperextension knee deformity is less frequent. A rigid extension deformity

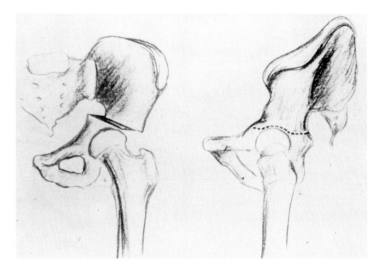

A

FIGURE 14.   (A) Chiari pelvic osteotomy. (B) Persistent left hip subluxation after Sharrad iliopsoas transfer. (C) Same patient as Figure 13B treated with a Chiari pelvic osteotomy.

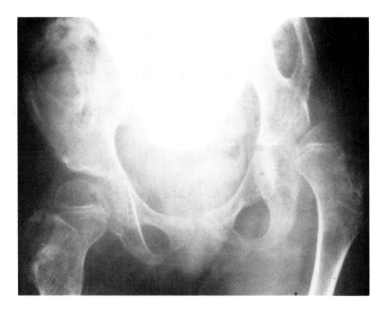

FIGURE 14B.

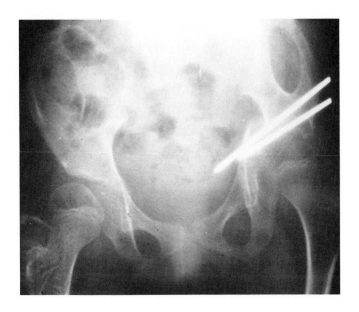

FIGURE 14C.

with no useful quadriceps power can be approached with surgical tenotomy or elongation of the patellar tendon and reticular releases at 6 to 8 years of age.

A quadricepsplasty or flexion osteotomy of the distal femur is rarely needed. Children with hyperextension contractures rarely become functional ambulators.[58]

Valgus deformity of the knee is usually due to iliotibial band contracture or fracture malunion. Appropriate release of the iliotibial band or distal femur osteotomy may be necessary in severe deformities.

XI. THE ANKLE

Valgus deformity of the hindfoot can occur at the subtalar joint or the ankle joint. In children with spina bifida, ankle valgus is most common, especially at the L4 to L5 neurosegmental level. Clinically, these children have a calcaneus foot with ankle valgus with excessive tendoachilles laxity and increased dorsiflexion associated with external tibial torsion. Hollingsworth[43] and Malhotra[67] noted in a radiologic study of ankle valgus in spina bifida that there was associated fibular shortening, lower tibial epiphyseal wedging, and valgus tilt of the ankle mortis. As can be expected, orthotic management of ankle valgus is fraught with difficulties (Figure 15).

The pathogenesis of ankle valgus in spina bifida is multifocal. In an extensive study, Dias concluded that fibular shortening was a result of soleus weakness.[20] Lateral tibial epiphyseal wedging is a result of abnormal joint

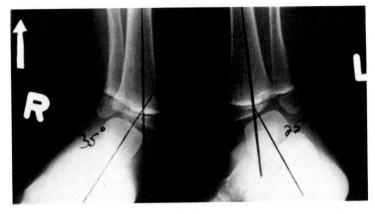

FIGURE 15.   L5 neurosegmental level. Bilateral ankle valgus at age 5+3.

forces applied to the distal tibial physis as a result of a shortened fibula and decreased lateral mortis support.

Before treatment is undertaken, it is essential that a thorough clinical assessment is performed: (1) the degree of contracture of the ankle dorsiflexors and evertors should be determined as these may need to be corrected and (2) the degree of valgus deformity in the subtalar joint should be assessed. Weight bearing roentgenogeous in the anteroposterior plane is essential to determine the degree of fibular shortening and the degree of wedging of the distal tibial epiphysis.

The treatment of ankle valgus encompasses several approaches. Foremost, the deformity should be recognized early and in children 8 to 12 years of age, medial distal tibial epiphyseal stapling can be helpful.[81] A calcaneofibular tendoachilles tenodesis, as described by Westin,[126] has been noted not only to prevent foot dorsiflexion but also to stimulate fibular growth. The calcaneotibial tenodesis[82] also has been very useful in preventing excessive foot dorsiflexion, but it will not correct talar tilt and this may have to be combined with a varus derotational supramalleolar osteotomy. As an adjunct, an anterior tibialis tendon transfer to the oscalcis through the interosseous membrane as a supplemental motor in the L4 to L5 functional patient.[7] In the late deformity, anterior and lateral ankle contractures will need simultaneous correction. In those patients with a combination of valgus deformity of the ankle and subtalar joint, Menelaus recommends both a supramalleolar tibial osteotomy and triple arthrodesis.[83]

XII. THE FOOT

A plantigrade foot that shoes and orthosis can fit comfortably is an expected goal in the management of myelomeningocele. Almost every foot deformity that can occur does occur in myelomeningocele either as a result of the disorder or of surgical management. The frequency of various foot deformities has been reported by many authors. Menelaus reported on 359 deformed feet in 190 children and 36% had varus or equinovarus deformities, 17% equinus, 3% cavovarus, 21% calcaneus, 6% calcaneovalgus, and 5% calcaneovara deformity.[77] Schafer and Dias noted that in 256 feet in 123 patients, only 23 feet had no deformities and that equinovarus and calcaneal deformities were the most common.[97]

Muscle imbalance is the primary cause of foot deformity and intra- and extrauterine positions adapted by the foot are secondary causes.

Several general observations about the management of foot deformity have been made by Menelaus:[77]

1. Fixed varus deformity requires complete correction by surgery.
2. Flail and mobile deformities requires appropriate orthoses.
3. Torseaxial and valgus deformities of the ankle joint are difficult to control with bracing and frequently require surgery.
4. Repeated operations are frequently necessary.
5. Subtalar, midtarsal, and triple arthrodeses are frequently helpful.[84] Ankle arthrodeses is not recommended.

A. Equinovarus Deformity

Although it is accepted that serial casting is seldom of definitive value in treating this deformity,[77,97,101] serial casting at birth to 3 months of age can be of some value in improving some of the deformity before surgery is undertaken. A closed achilles tenotomy can be performed when it is apparent that further correction cannot be achieved. A thorough posteromedial soft tissue release is generally necessary between the ages of 4 months and 1 year of age. A portion of the posterior tibialis tendon should be excised and those tendons that are not functional should be sectioned as part of the release. If the equinovarus deformity cannot be corrected by radical posteromedial release alone, then calcaneocuboid excision fusion,[33] Lichtblau procedure,[56] or cuboid deconcellation should be performed.

Tendon transfers have not been helpful in any consistent fashion in equinovarus deformity in myelomeningocele. Persistent residual deformities may require additional surgery. Recurrent equinus deformity may require posterior release with tendoachilles tenotomy. Residual heel varus may require a Dwyer osteotomy of the oscalcis but should be performed between 4 to 8 years of age.

Talectomy can be utilized as a salvage procedure for severe and rigid deformity seen late in the older child that has not responded to radical soft tissue releases.[21] Menelaus reports that the best age for talectomy is between the ages of 1 and 5 years. Successful results have been reported by Shark and Ames[105] in 75% of feet. The surgery was done between 2 and 9 years of age. Cuboid excision in conjunction with talectomy has been advocated by Carroll and Dias to correct forefoot adduction.

Distal tibial rotational osteotomy may need to be considered if persistent

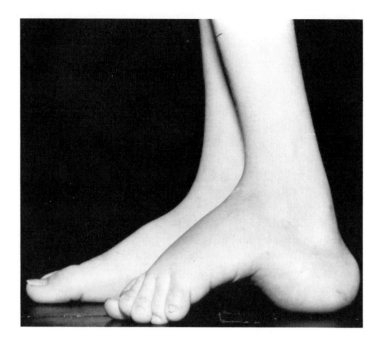

FIGURE 16.   Talipes calcaneus L5 neurosegmental level. Note cavus forefoot.

beyond 4 to 5 years of age to correct persistent internal tibial torsion which may be associated with a varus foot.

In the late rigid equinovarus deformity in children 11 to 14 years of age or older, triple arthrodesis may be indicated. All muscle imbalance needs to be corrected at the time of the fusion, however, or recurrent deformity can occur.[23,77]

B. Calcaneus Deformity

Calcaneus deformity is due to activity of the anterior compartment muscles in the absence of calf muscle activity (Figure 16). Although uncommon, unbalanced overactivity of the tibialis anterior and tibialis posterior can lead to calcaneovarus deformity. The most common deformity, however, is calcaneovalgus.

Calcaneus deformity, if untreated, leads to abnormal pressure on the heel with frequent skin breakdown and poor shoe wear.

External tibial torsion is often associated with hindfoot valgus. Correction of the foot valgus without correction of the external tibial torsion will lead to recurrence.

Children should be treated orthotically and muscle power assessed up to 1 to 5 years of age. At 5 years of age, the anterior tibialis can be transferred through the interosseous membrane to the oscalcis along with sectioning of the

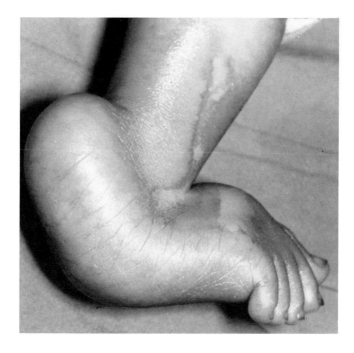

FIGURE 17.   Vertical talus.

toe extensors.[9] If the anterior tibialis is weak or spastic, then an achilles tenodesis to the tibia or fibula is recommended. In the latter case, anterior ankle capsulotomy will be necessary.

In patients with severe calcaneovalgus deformity, the treatment of the calcaneal deformity will require supplemental correction of the valgus deformity of the subtalar joint. In this instance, a subtalar arthrodesis between the ages of 3 and 10 years of age[30] or a triple arthrodesis over the age of 11 to 15 years will need to be considered. Nicol et al.[83] have reported excellent results by combining triple arthrodesis and supramalleolar tibial rotational osteotomy.

C. Paralytic Convex Pes Valgus (Vertical Tallus)

Paralytic convex pes valgus is the same as the congenital variety but less rigid (Figure 17). It is caused by strong evertors and dorsiflexors of the foot that overpower the paralytic tibialis posterior.[24] A one-stage procedure that combines soft tissue releases and tendon transfers has given satisfactory results.[23,25] Surgical correction should be considered early between the ages of 6 and 18 months of age.

A medial incision is utilized for anterior and posterior subtalar capsulotomies as well as posterior ankle capsulotomy. The anterior tendons on the dorsum of the foot are divided and the dislocated talonavicular joint is reduced and fixed with a Kirschner wire. A lateral incision is used to release the calcaneocuboid and the lateral aspect of the subtalar joint. The reduced calcaneocuboid and subtalar joints are also fixed with Kirschner wires.

The above procedures can be combined with either transfer of the anterior tibialis tendon into the talar neck[122] or transfer of the peroneus brevis across the posterior aspect of the tibia into the tendon sheath of the tibialis posterior and inserted into the navicular.[25,77] If a tendon transfer is not possible, then the subtalar joint can be stabilized with a subtalar fusion[77] as described by Dennyson et al.[18] After reduction and stabilization of the talonavicular, subtalar joints and calcaneocuboid joints are accomplished and a tendoachilles lengthening is performed. Nonweight bearing long leg casting is recommended for 4 months.[23,25]

D. Equinus Deformity

Paralytic equinus deformity can be prevented with a combination of physiotherapy and the use of an ankle foot orthosis (AFO) routinely. More rigid equinus deformities may require percutaneous tenotomy of the tendoachilles or posterior capsulotomy. Consistent use of an articulated ankle foot orthosis with a 90° plantar flexion stop will minimize recurrences.

E. Pes Planovalgus Deformity

Although this deformity is not usually a problem in myelomeningocele, some patients will have difficulty with pressure sores over the talar head with orthotic wear. A subtalar fusion can be considered[18] or a sliding calcaneal osteotomy[97,121] if surgical correction is desirable. In the child over age 11 to 14, a triple arthrodesis is useful as recommended by Menelaus.[77]

F. Claw Toe Deformity

Claw toe deformity is usually seen in children with a sacral neurosegmental level. Tenodesis of the flexor halluces longers to the plantar aspect of the proximal phalanx is useful in correction of clawing of the hallux.[102] Clawing of the lateral four toes can be corrected by the Girdlestone-Taylor tendon transfer.[119]

REFERENCES

1. **Abraham, E., Verinder, D. G. R., and Sharrard, W. J. W.,** The treatment of flexion contracture of the knee in myelomeningocele, *J. Bone Jt. Sur.,* 59B, 433, 1977.
2. **Asher, M. and Olson, J.,** Does hip dislocation and subluxation affect ambulation in the patient with spina bifida aptica?, *Orthop. Trans.,* 5, p. 4, 1981.
3. **Allen, B. L., Jr.,** The operative treatment of myelomeningocele spinal deformity, *Orthop. Clin. N. Am.,* 10(4), 845, 1979.
4. **Allen, B. L., Jr. and Ferguson, R. L.,** The place for segmental instrumentation in the treatment of spine deformity, *Orthop. Trans.,* 6(1), 21, 1982.

5. **Banta, J. V. and Hamada, J. S.,** Natural history of the kyphotic deformity in myelomeningocele, *J. Bone Jt. Surg.,* 58A, 279, 1976.

6. **Banta, J. V., Whiteman, S., Dyck, R. M., Hartleip, D., and Gilbert, D.,** Fifteen year review of myelodysplasia, *J. Bone Jt. Surg.,* 58A, 726, 1976.

7. **Banta, J. V., Sutherland, D. H., and Wyatt, M.,** Anterior tibial transfer to the oscalcis with achilles tenodesis for calcaneal deformity in myelomeningocele, *J. Pediatr. Orthop.,* 1, 125, 1981.

8. **Barden, G. A., Meyer, L. C., and Stelling, F. H.,** Myelodysplastics: fate of those followed for twenty years or more, *J. Bone Jt. Surg.,* 57A, 643, 1975.

9. **Bliss, D. G. and Menelaus, M. B.,** The results of transfer of the tibialis anterior to the heel in patients who have myelomeningocele, *J. Bone Jt. Surg.,* 68A(8), 1258, 1986.

10. **Brock, D. J. and Sutcliffe, R. G.,** Alphafetoprotein in the antenatal diagnosis of anencephaly and spina bifida, *Lancet,* 2, 197, 1972.

11. **Bunch, W. H. and Hakala, M. W.,** Iliopsoas transfers in children with myelomeningocele, *J. Bone Jt. Surg.,* 66A, 124, 1984.

12. **Bunch, W. H.,** The Milwaukee brace in paralytic scoliosis, *Clin. Orthop.,* 110, 63, 1975.

13. **Bunch, W. H., Scarff, T. B., and Drouch, V.,** Progressive neurological loss in myelomeningocele patients, *Orthop. Trans.,* 7(1), 185, 1983.

14. **Carr, T. L.,** The orthopaedic aspects of one hundred cases of spina bifida, *Postgrad. Med. J.,* 32, 201, 1956.

15. **Carter, C. O. and Evans, K.,** Children of adult survivors with spina bifida aptica, *Lancet,* 2, 924, 1973.

16. **Chiari, K.,** Medical displacement osteotomy of the pelvis, *Clin. Orthop.,* 98, 55, 1974.

17. **Cruess, R. L. and Turner, N. S.,** Paralysis of hip abductor muscles in spina bifida: results of treatment by the Mustard procedure, *J. Bone Jt. Surg.,* 52A, 1364, 1970.

18. **Dennyson, W. G. and Fulford, G. E.,** Subtalar arthrodesis by cancellous grafts and metallic internal fixation, *J. Bone Jt. Surg.,* 58B, 507, 1976.

19. **Dias, L. S. and Hill, J. A.,** Evaluation of treatment of hip subluxation in myelomeningocele by intertrochanteric varus derotation femoral osteotomy, *Orthop. Clin. North Am.,* 11, 31, 1980.

20. **Dias, L. S.,** Ankle valgus in children with myelomeningocele, *Div. Med. Child Neurol.,* 20, 627, 1978.

21. **Diaz, L. S. and Stern, L. S.,** Talectomy in the treatment of resistant talipes equinovarus deformity in myelomeningocele and arthrogryposis, *J. Pediatr. Orthop.,* 7, 39, 1981.

22. **Doran, P. A. and Guthkelch, A. N.,** Studies on spina bifida. IV. The frequency and extent of the paralysis, *J. Neurol. Neurosurg. Psychiat.,* 26, 545, 1963.

23. **Drennan, J. C.,** *Orthopaedic Management of Neuromuscular Disorder,* Lippincott, New York, 1983.

24. **Drennan, J. C. and Sharrard, W. J. W.,** The pathologic anatomy of convex pes valgus, *J. Bone Jt. Surg.,* 53B, 455, 1971.

25. **Drennan, J. C.,** Management of myelomeningocele foot deformities in infancy and early childhood, *Am. Acad. Ortho. Surg. Instruc. Course Lect.,* 25, 82, 1976.

26. **Drennan, J. C.,** Orthotic management of the myelomeningocele spine, *Dev. Med. Child. Neurol.,* 18(Suppl. 37), 97, 1976.

27. **Drennan, J. C.,** The role of muscles in the development of human lumbar kyphosis, *Dev. Med. Child. Neurol.,* 12, 33, 1970.

28. **Drummond, D., Breed, A. L., and Narechanea, R.,** Relationship of spine deformity and pelvic obliquity on sitting pressure distributions and decubitus ulceration, *J. Pediatr. Orthop.,* 5(4), 396, 1985.

29. **Dunn, H. K.,** Kyphosis of myelodysplasia — operative treatment based on pathophysiology, *Orthop. Trans.,* 7(1), 19, 1983.

30. **Edwards, E. R. and Menelaus, M.,** Reverse clubfoot — rigid and recalcitrant talipes calcaneovalgus, *J. Bone Jt. Surg.,* 69B(2), 330, 1987.

31. **Eggers, G. W. N.,** Transplantation of hamstring tendons to femoral condyles in order to improve hip extension and to decrease knee flexion in cerebral spastic paralysis, *J. Bone Jt. Surg.,* 34A, 827, 1952.

32. **Elias, E. R. and Siber, M. W.,** Tethered cord syndrome, *Div. Med. Child Neurol.,* 30(5), (Suppl. 57), 26, 1988.

33. **Evans, D.,** Relapsed clubfoot, *J. Bone Jt. Surg.,* 43B, 722, 1961.

34. **Eyring, E. J., Wanken, J. J., and Sayers, M. P.,** Spinal osteotomy for kyphosis in myelomeningocele, *Clin. Orthop.,* 88, 24, 1972.

35. **Feiwell, E., Sakai, D., and Blatt, T.,** The effect of hip reduction on function in patients with myelomeningocele: potential gains and hazards of surgical treatment, *J. Bone Jt. Surg.,* 60A, 169, 1978.

36. **Feiwell, E.,** Surgery of the hip in myelomeningocele as related to adult goals, *Clin. Orthop.,* 148, 87, 1980.

37. **Forrest, D.,** Spina Bifida. Practice and ethical considerations in its treatment, *Mod. Med.,* 17, 108, 1974.

38. **Hall, J. E. and Martin, R.,** The Natural History of Spine Deformity in myelomeningocele. A study of 130 patients, *Proc. Can. Orthop. Assoc.,* Bermuda, June 1970.

39. **Hall, J. E. and Poitra, B.,** The management of kyphosis in patients with myelomeningocele, *Clin. Orthop.,* 128, 33, 1977.

40. **Hayes, J. T. and Gross, H. P.,** Orthopaedic implications of myelodysplasia, *JAMA,* 184, 762, 1963.

41. **Heydermann, J. S. and Gillespie, R.,** Management of myelomeningocele kyphosis in the older child by kyphectomy and segmental spinal instrumentation, *Spine,* 12(1), 37, 1987.

42. **Hoffer, M. M., Feiwell, E., Perry, J., and Bonnett, C.,** Functional ambulation in patients with myelomeningocele, *J. Bone Jt. Surg.,* 55A, 137, 1973.

43. **Hollingsworth, R. P.,** An X-ray study of valgus ankles in spina bifida children with valgoid flat foot deformity, *Proc. R. Soc. Med.,* 68, 481, 1975.

44. **Hoppenfeld, S.,** Congenital kyphosis in myelomeningocele, *J. Bone Jt. Surg.,* 49B, 276, 1967.

45. **Hostler, S. L.,** Development of the infant with myelomeningocele, *Am. Acad. Orthop. Surg. Instruct. Course Lect.,* 25, 70, 1976.

46. **Huff, C. W. and Ramsey, P. L.,** Myelodysplasia: the influence of the quadriceps and hip abductor muscles for ambulatory function and stability of the hips, *J. Bone Jt. Surg.,* 60A, 432, 1978.

47. **Hughes, W. A. and Dias, L. S.,** Scoliosis in myelomeningocele: the role of tethered cord and hydromyelia, *Div. Med Child Neurol.,* 30(5), (Suppl. 57), 26, 1988.

48. **Hull, W. J., Moe, J. H., Lai, C., and Winter, R. B.,** The surgical treatment of spinal deformities in myelomeningocele, *J. Bone Jt. Surg.,* 57A, 1767, 1974.

49. **Hunt, G. M., Walpole, L., Gelave, J., and Gairdner, D.,** Predictive factors in open myelomeningocele with special reference to sensory level, *Br. Med. J.,* 4, 197, 1973.

50. **Jackson, R. D., Padgett, R. S., and Donovan, M. M.,** Iliopsoas muscle transfer in myelodysplasia, *J. Bone Jt. Surg.,* 61A, 40, 1969.

51. **Jones, G. B.,** Paralytic dislocation of the hip, *J. Bone Jt. Surg.,* 36B, 375, 1954.

52. **Kupka, J., Rey, O. T., Geddes, N., and Carroll, N. C.,** Developmental landmarks in spina bifida, *Orthop. Clin. N. Am.,* 9(1), 97, 1978.

53. **Lawrence, K. M.,** The recurrence risk in spina bifida aptica and anencephaly, *Div. Med. Child Neurol.,* 23(Suppl. 20), 1969.

54. **Laurence, K. M.,** The natural history of spina bifida aptica. Detailed analysis of 407 cases, *Arch. Dis. Child.,* 39, 41, 1964.

55. **Laurence, K. and Tew, B. J.,** Natural history of spina bifida aptica and cranium bifidum apticum. Major central nervous system malformations in South Wales, *Arch. Dis. Child.,* 46, 127, 1971.

56. **Lichtblau, S.,** A medial and lateral release operation for a club foot, *J. Bone Jt. Surg.,* 55A, 1377, 1973.

57. **Lindseth, R. E.,** Posterior iliac osteotomy for fixed pelvic obliquity, *J. Bone Jt. Surg.,* 60A, 17, 1978.

58. **Lindseth, R. E.,** Treatment of the lower extremity in children paralyzed by Myelomeningocele, *Am. Acad. Orthop. Surg. Instruc. Course Lect.,* 25, 76, 1976.

59. **Lindseth, R. E. and Stelzer, L.,** Vertebral excision for kyphosis in children with myelomeningocele, *J. Bone Jt. Surg.,* 61A, 699, 1979.

60. **Lloyd-Roberts, C. G., Williams, D. I., and Braddock, G. T. F.,** Pelvic osteotomy in the treatment of ectapia vesical, *J. Bone Jt. Surg.,* 41B, 754, 1959.

61. **Lorber, J.,** Results of treatment of myelomeningocele, *Div. Med. Child Neurol.,* 13, 279, 1971.

62. **Lorber, J.,** Selective treatment of myelomeningocele: to treat or not to treat, *Pediatrics,* 53, 307, 1974.

63. **Lowman, C. L.,** Lateral fascial transplant for controlling a gluteus medius limp, *Physiother. Rev.,* 27, 355, 1947.

64. **Luque, E. R.,** Kyphosis and lordosis, correction and production, *Orthop. Trans.,* 5(1), 16, 1981.

65. **Mackel, J. L. and Lindseth, R. E.,** Scoliosis in myelodysplasia, *J. Bone Jt. Surg.,* 57A, 1031, 1975.

66. **Maguire, C. D., Winter, R. B., Mayfield, J. K., and Erickson, D. L.,** Hemimyelodysplasia: a report of 10 cases, *J. Pediatr. Orthop.,* 2(1), 9, 1982.

67. **Malhotra, D., Puri, R., and Owen, R.,** Valgus deformity of the ankle in children with spina bifida aperta, *J. Bone Jt. Surg.,* 66B, 381, 1984.

68. **Marchetti, P. G.,** End fusions in the treatment of some progressing or severe scoliosis in childhood or early adolescence, *Proc. 12th Scoliosis Res. Soc. Meet.,* Hong Kong, October 24 to 27, 1977.

69. **Mayfield, J. K.,** Spine deformity in myelomeningocele, in *The Pediatric Spine,* Thieme, New York, 1985, 368.

70. **Mayfield, J. K.,** Severe spine deformity in myelodysplasia and sacral agenesis — an aggressive surgical approach, *Spine,* 6(5), 498, 1981.

71. **Mayfield, J. K. and King, H.,** Congenital lumbar kyphosis — an alternative instrumentation system, *18th Annu. Scoliosis Res. Soc. Meet.,* New Orleans, September 28 to October 1, 1983.

72. **Mayfield, J. K., Erkkila, J. C., and Winter, R. B.,** Spine deformity subsequent to acquired childhood spinal cord injury, *J. Bone Jt. Surg.,* 63A(9), 1401, 1981.

73. **Mazur, J. M., Stillwell, A., and Mandous, M.,** The significance of spasticity in the upper and lower limbs in myelomeningocele, *J. Bone Jt. Surg.,* 68B(2), 213, 1986.

74. **McKibben, B.,** The use of splintage in the management of paralytic dislocation of the hip in spina bifida cystica, *J. Bone Jt. Surg.,* 55B, 163, 1973.

75. **McMaster, M.,** Anterior and posterior instrumentation and fusion of thoracolumbar scoliosis due to myelomeningocele, *J. Bone Jt. Surg.,* 69B(1), 20, 1987.

76. **McMaster, M.,** The long term results of kyphectomy and spinal stabilization in children with myelomeningocele spine, 13(4), 4, 1988.

77. **Menelaus, M. B.,** *The Orthopaedic Management of Spina Bifida Cystica,* Churchill Livingstone, Edinburgh, 1980.

78. **Menelaus, M. B.,** The hip in myelomeningocele, *J. Bone Jt. Surg.,* 58B, 448, 1976.

79. **Moe, J. K., Winter, R. B., Bradford, D. S., and Lonstein, J. E.,** *Scoliosis and Other Spinal Deformities,* W. B. Saunders, Philadelphia, 1987.

80. **Moe, J. H., Cummins, J. L., Winter, R. B., Groesler, L., and Bradford, D. S.,** Harrington instrumentation without fusion combined with the Milwaukee brace for difficult scoliosis problems in young children, *Orthop. Trans.,* 3(1), 59, 1979.

81. **Moore, D. W., Raycroft, J. F., Loyer, R. E., and Paul, S. W.,** The treatment of disabling foot and ankle valgus in myelodysplastic children, *Proc. Am. Acad. Orthop. Surg.,* Dallas, 1978.

82. **Mustard, W. T. and McDonald, G.,** The Gallie tenodesis, *Can. Med. Assoc. J.,* 75, 271, 1956.

83. **Nicol, R. O. and Menelaus, M. D.,** Correction of combined tibial torsion and valgus deformity of the foot, *J. Bone Jt. Surg.,* 65B, 641, 1983.

84. **Olney, B. W. and Menelaus, M. B.,** Triple arthrodesis of the foot in spina bifida patients, *J. Bone Jt. Surg.,* 70B(2), 234, 1988.

85. **O'Phelan, E. H.,** Iliac osteotomy in extrophy of the bladder, *J. Bone Jt. Surg.,* 45A 1409, 1963.

86. **Osebold, W. R., Mayfield, J. K., Winter, R. B., and Moe, J. H.,** Surgical treatment of paralytic scoliosis associated with myelomeningocele, *J. Bone Jt. Surg.,* 64A, 841, 1982.

87. **Parker, B. and Waltor, R.,** Posterior psoas transfer and hip instability in lumbar myelomeningocele, *J. Bone Jt. Surg.,* 57B, 53, 1975.

88. **Parsch, K. and Manner, G.,** Prevention and treatment of knee problems in children with spina bifida, *Div. Med. Child Neurol.,* 18(6), (Suppl. 37), 114, 1976.

89. **Paul, S. W.,** Spinal problems in myelomeningocele — orthotic principles, *Prost. Orthot. Int.,* 1, 30, 1977.

90. **Pemberton, P. A.,** Pericapsular osteotomy of the ilium for treatment of congenital subluxation and dislocation of the hip, *J. Bone Jt. Surg.,* 47A, 65, 1965.

91. **Piggott, H.,** The natural history of scoliosis in myelodysplasia, *J. Bone Jt. Surg.,* 62B(1), 54, 1980.

92. **Pillard, D., Massy, P., and Taussing, G.,** The hip in myelomeningocele, *Orthop. Trans.,* 5, 61, 1981.

93. **Raycroft, J. E. and Curtis, B. H.,** *Spinal Curvature in Myelomeningocele; Natural History and Etiology,* C. V. Mosby, St. Louis, 1972.

94. **Record, R. G. and McKeown, T.,** Congenital malformations of the central nervous system: a survey of 930 cases, *Br. J. Prev. Soc. Med.,* 3, 183, 1949.

95. **Rivard, C. H., Legendre, P., Marton, D., and Poitras, B.,** Iliopsoas muscle transfer in low-lumbar myelomeningocele: parameters associated with a stable hip, *J. Bone Jt. Surg.,* 67B, 333, 1985.

96. **Salter, R. B.,** Innominate osteotomy in the treatment of congenital dislocation and subluxation of the hip, *J. Bone Jt. Surg.,* 43B, 518, 1961.

97. **Schafer, M. F. and Dias, L. S.,** *Myelomeningocele, Orthopaedic Treatment,* Williams & Wilkins, Baltimore, 1983.

98. **Sharrard, W. J. W.,** The segmental innervation of the lower limb muscles in man, *Ann. R. Coll. Surg.,* 35, 106, 1964.

99. **Sharrard, W. J. W.,** Congenital paralytic dislocation of the hip in children with myelomeningocele, *J. Bone Jt. Surg.,* 41B, 622, 1959.

100. **Sharrard, W. J. W.,** Long term follow-up of posterior transplant for paralytic dislocation of the hip, *J. Bone Jt. Surg.,* 5LB, 779, 1970.

101. **Sharrard, W. J. W. and Grossfield, I.,** The management of deformity and paralysis of the foot in myelomeningocele, *J. Bone Jt. Surg.,* 50B, 456, 1968.

102. **Sharrard, W. J. W. and Smith, T. W. D.,** Tenodesis of flexor hallucis longus for paralytic clawing of the hallux in childhood, *J. Bone Jt. Surg.,* 58B, 274, 1976.

103. **Sharrard, W. J. W.,** *The Kyphotic and Lordotic Spine in Myelomeningocele,* C. V. Mosby, St. Louis, 1972.

104. **Sharrard, W. J. W.,** Spinal osteotomy for congenital kyphosis in myelomeningocele, *J. Bone Jt. Surg.,* 50B, 466, 1968.

105. **Shark, H. H. and Ames, M. D.,** Talectomy in the treatment of the myelomeningocele patient, *Clin. Orthop.,* 110, 218, 1975.

106. **Shark, H. H., Melchionni, J., and Smith, R.,** Treatment vs. non-treatment of hip dislocations in ambulatory patients with myelomeningocele, *Dev. Med. Child Neurol.,* 30(5), (Suppl. 57), 5, 1988.

163

107. **Shurleff, D. B., Menelaus, M. B., Staheli, L. T., Chow, D. E., Larners, B. S., Stillwell, A., and Wolf, L. S.,** Natural history of flexion deformity of the hip in myelodysplasia, *J. Pediatr. Orthop.,* 6(6), 666, 1986.

108. **Shurleff, D. B., Bourney, R., Gordon, L. H., and Livermore, N.,** Myelodysplasia: the natural history of kyphosis and scoliosis. A preliminary report, *Dev. Med. Child Neurol.,* 18(Suppl. 37), 126, 1976.

109. **Siebens, A., Hohf, J., Sugel, E., and Scribner, N.,** Suspension of certain patients from their ribs, *Johns Hopkins Med. J.,* 130, 26, 1972.

110. **Simpson, D.,** Congenital malformations of the nervous system, *Med. J. Aust.,* 1, 700, 1976.

111. **Smith, G. K. and Smith, E. D.,** Selection for treatment in spina bifida cystica, *Br. Med. J.,* 4, 189, 1973.

112. **Stack, G. D. and Drummond, M.,** Results of selective early operations in myelomeningocele, *Arch. Dis. Child.,* 48, 676, 1973.

113. **Stack, G. D.,** Myelomeningocele: the changing approach to treatment, in *Recent Advances in Pediatric Surgery,* Churchill Livingstone, London, 1975, 73.

114. **Stack, G. D. and Baber, G. C.,** The neurological involvement of the lower limbs in myelomeningocele, *Dev. Med. Child Neurol.,* 9, 732, 1967.

115. **Steele, H. H.,** Triple osteotomy of the innominate bone, *J. Bone Jt. Surg.,* 55A, 343, 1973.

116. **Stillwell, A. and Menelaus, M. B.,** Walking ability in mature patients with spina bifida, *J. Pediatr. Orthop.,* 3(2), 184, 1983.

117. **Sriram, K., Bobechko, W. P., and Hall, J. E.,** Surgical management of spinal deformities in spina bifida, *J. Bone Jt. Surg.,* 54B, 666, 1972.

118. **Sullivan, J. A. and Conner, S.,** Segmental spinal instrumentation by laminar wiring, *Orthop. Trans.,* 5(1), 17, 1981.

119. **Taylor, R. G.,** The treatment of claw toes by multiple transfers of flexor into extensor tendons, *J. Bone Jt. Surg.,* 66B, 381, 1984.

120. **Thomas, L. I., Thompson, T. C. and Straub, L. R.,** Transplantation of the external oblique muscle for abductor paralysis, *J. Bone Jt. Surg.,* 332A, 207, 1950.

121. **Trieshmann, H., Millis, M., Hall, J., and Watts, H.,** Sliding calcaneal osteotomy for treatment of hindfoot deformity, *Orthop. Trans.,* 4, 305, 1980.

122. **Walker, G. and Cheong-leen, P.,** Surgical management of paralytic vertical talus in myelomeningocele, *Dev. Med. Child Neurol.,* 15(6), (Suppl. 29), 112, 1973.

123. **Wallace, H. M., Baumgartner, L., and Rich, J.,** Congenital malformations and birth injuries in New York City, *Pediatrics,* 12, 525, 1953.

124. **Weiner, L. S., Burke, S. W., and Root, L.,** The use of MRI in myelodysplasia, *Dev. Med. Child Neurol.,* 30(5), (Suppl. 57), 27, 1988.

125. **Weisl, H., Fairclough, J. A., and Jones, D. G.,** Stabilization of the hip in myelomeningocele — comparison of posterior iliopsoas transfer and varus rotation osteotomy, *J. Bone Jt. Surg.,* 70B(1), 29, 1988.

126. **Westin, G. W. and Defiore, R. J.,** Tenodesis of the tendo-achilles to the fibula for a paralytic calcaneus deformity, *J. Bone Jt. Surg.,* 56A, 1541, 1975.

127. **Winston, K., Hall, J., Johnson, D., and Micheli, L.,** Acute elevation of intracranial pressure following transection of non-functional spinal cord, *Clin. Orthop.,* 128, 41, 1977.

128. **Winter, R. B. and Moe, J. H.,** Modern orthotics for spinal deformities, *Clin. Orthop.,* 126, 76, 1977.

129. **Winter, R. B., Moe, J. H., and Eilers, V. E.,** Congenital scoliosis. A study of 234 patients treated and untreated. I. Natural history, *J. Bone Jt. Surg.,* 50A, 1, 1968.

130. **Wissinger, H. A., Tumer, Y., and Donaldson, W. F.,** Posterior iliopsoas transfer: a treatment for some myelodysplastic hips, *Orthopaedics,* 3, 865, 1980.

Chapter 7

THE USE OF ORTHOTICS IN THE TREATMENT OF MYELOMENINGOCELE

R. Craig Pomatto

TABLE OF CONTENTS

The orthotic care of the multiply handicapped child is one of the most challenging and rewarding treatment regimes encountered by the clinical orthotist.
The myelomeningocele affected child frequently presents us with a multiply
handicapped patient capable of developing average to above average intellectual and perceptual motor skills.[1-5]

Among the factors that influence the development of these skills are the
child's ability to interact with and manipulate their environment. The extent to
which these abilities are encouraged to develop can have a positive influence
on the child's feelings of self-esteem and their eventual integration into society
as functional adults capable of managing a family and a career.

Integral to the development of a healthy self-esteem is the child's ability to
interact with their environment in as near normal a fashion as is physiologically
possible. It is the intention of the cooperative efforts of the orthopedist,
physical therapist, and orthotist to parallel the major milestones of development as closely as possible. The goals of sitting, crawling, standing, and
walking in their appropriate chronological sequence is the therapeutic emphasis of current orthotic care.

Due to the complex multisystem involvement associated with a diagnosis of
myelomeningocele, a multidisciplinary approach to the treatment of this handicap is vital.[4] The efforts of the clinic team must be carefully coordinated in
order to attain the type of results that enhance the child's developmental
potential. The treatment goals established by the orthopedist can be difficult to
achieve when they are hindered by ill-fitting or out-of-date orthotic devices and
inadequate physical therapy modalities.

The past 20 years of research and development in the field of orthotics have
provided us with dramatically improved materials and the clinical framework
in which to apply these new materials. From the vantage point of current
technology, we are able to see prior art as a study of compromises; function at
the expense of cosmesis and durability at the expense of energy efficiency.
Advances in thermoplastic technology now allow us to develop lightweight
orthotic devices with superior biomechanical control, improved cosmesis, and
durability without the previously significant penalties to our patient's often
limited energy reservoir. The inadequacies inherent in conventional double
upright lower extremity orthosis are well understood; their principal weakness
is in the foot-shoe interface. A leather shoe, regardless of the care utilized in
fitting it, is inadequate to control the mediolateral forces crossing the subtalar
joint of the flail foot. Leather is a highly malleable material, especially when
wet. In a short period of time, even with the use of a T-strap, it will deform in
the direction of the pathological motion. Attempts to accommodate the resultant deformity with shoe wedging in order to balance floor reaction forces are
questionable.[6] Once the attempt to maintain normal subtalar positioning is
compromised, the pathomechanical forces arising from the malpositioned
ankle complex are transmitted proximally, creating abnormal loads at the knee
and hip.

Current concepts in the fabrication of total contact plastic ankle foot orthosis are providing us with answers to the limitations of conventional metal and leather lower extremity orthotic systems. Prior to our discussion of these systems we review the materials, fabrication techniques, and fitting criteria utilized in current thermoplastic and carbon fiber technology.

I. CURRENT CONCEPTS IN FABRICATION AND FITTING

The application of polypropylene and polyethylene thermoplastic fabrication technologies to the field of orthotics was responsible for significant advances in our ability to deliver corrective forces to the body. The use of thermoplastics in brace fabrication necessitated the creation of a positive mold over which these plastics would then be vacuumformed (Figure 3).

A negative impression is taken of the patient's extremity and then filled with plaster of Paris to create the positive model. This positive model allows the orthotist to cast the extremity in as anatomically correct a position as possible and then further improve this correction, if desirable, during the process of preparing the positive model for vacuumforming (Figures 1 and 2). The procedure enhances the control of pathological alignment anomalies by allowing the orthotist to capture and correct the affected extremity in a three-dimensional fashion.

Prior to the development of these fabrication techniques, all morphological data were taken from the patient in the form of measurements and tracings of the patient's extremity. Gathering data from a three-dimensional object in a two-dimensional fashion results in a significant loss of information as compared to the impression and mold fabrication techniques described previously.

The use of conventional metal and leather technologies to apply corrective forces to the body usually results in highly focused areas of pressure distribution. For example, the use of a T-strap to correct ankle valgus deformities applies the greatest part of the corrective force just proximal to the medial malleolus. In most cases, the force necessary to effect a reasonable correction cannot be tolerated by the patient, resulting in a loss of correction either through patient intolerance or by the gradual deformation of the leather over a short period of time.

Plastic fabrication techniques allow us to distribute these corrective forces over a greater tissue area, resulting in a total contact interface between the body and the orthosis. This interface is the most significant gain derived from modern plastics technology. The preparation of the model is, in essence, the decision making process whereby the orthotist directs the corrective force to pressure tolerant tissues while ensuring that the same forces are prevented from occurring over pressure-intolerant tissues. A total contact plastic orthosis fabricated from a well-modified and corrected impression will follow closely the anatomical contours of the body with no discernible gapping except that

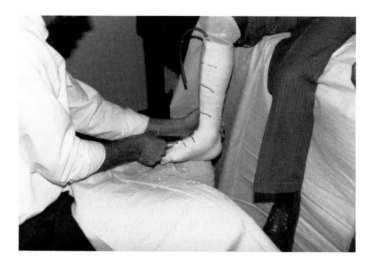

FIGURE 1. AFO impression procedure.

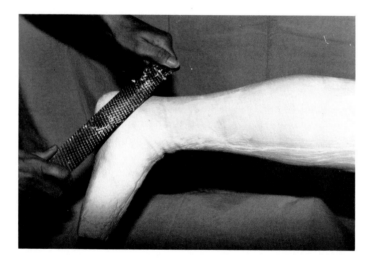

FIGURE 2. Mold modification process.

which is necessary to protect pressure intolerant tissues (Figures 4 and 5). An orthosis that exhibits excessive gapping is not delivering the optimal biomechanical forces to the body. In a correctly fitting, total contact plastic orthosis, there should be very little room for circumferential growth. Growth adjustments can be accomplished, to a limited degree, by reheating and expanding the orthosis to the desired size.

Durability and rigidity of plastic orthoses were, at one time, difficult to

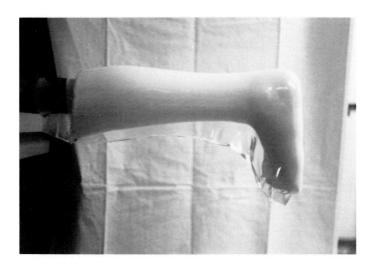

FIGURE 3. Vacuumforming process.

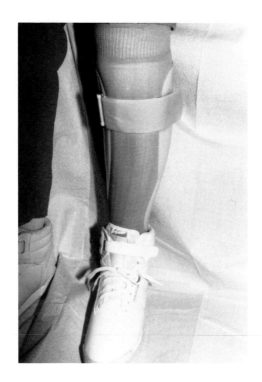

FIGURE 4. Total contact AFO.

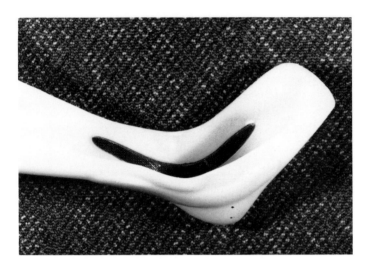

FIGURE 5. Carbon fiber reinforcing.

achieve. As these techniques were being developed, polypropylene was, and still is in certain instances, the material of choice due to the superior rigidity inherent in this material. However, polypropylene is susceptible to stress fracturing after repeated cyclic loading normally encountered during gait. In answer to this compromise of rigidity at the expense of durability, a blend of polypropylene and polyethylene (a more flexible thermoplastic) was developed and marketed under the name of copolymer polypropylene. Copolymer polypropylene can tolerate extensive cyclic loading without fatigue but it does so at the expense of the rigidity found in unblended polypropylene. This deficiency has recently been answered by the incorporation of carbon graphite composite reinforcing materials at areas of high stress where additional rigidity is warranted (Figure 6). This type of rigidity is highly desirable when ambulating the flail foot ankle complex normally associated with myelomeningocele.

II. THE ORTHOTIC TREATMENT
OF MYELOMENINGOCELE

As previously stated, the primary goals during the first years of life are to assist the child in attaining typical developmental milestones of sitting, crawling, standing, and walking. Many variables affect the degree to which the infant will ultimately succeed in developing these skills. Important among these are the degree of the neural involvement, the presence of hydrocephalus, the condition of the shunt, the home environment, and the socioeconomic status of the family. In addition, the extent to which the infant has been

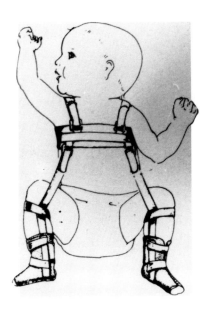

FIGURE 6. Pavlic harness.

hospitalized and his ability to interact with and be stimulated by his environment are significant to the development of these skills.[1-3,5-8]

In assisting the infant in achieving a developmental course as near to normal as possible, we hope to provide them with an environment conducive to the subsequent development of normal intellectual, psychosocial, and perceptual-motor skills.

Essential to the ability of the infant to develop and explore the environment are the preservation of joint range of motion, stable joint approximation, the prevention and correction of significant spinal deformity, and to either create or maintain a plantargrade foot.[18]

The role of the orthotist during the infant's first year of life is to assist the orthopedic surgeon in attaining the previously stated goals through positioning the infant in such a manner that significant deformity is prevented from occurring or, after surgical intervention, from recurring. Positioning the infant during the first month of life is directed at preventing hip subluxation and to avoid any pressure on the feet that would tend to aggravate any foot deformities.

The infant is placed prone in the bed with a pad between his legs to maintain his hips in abduction, thus counteracting the tendency to sublux. A Pavlic harness is useful as it allows easy diaper changing and perineal care without the removal of the orthosis (Figure 7). As the infant grows, the use of a COH hip abduction splint may be of value as it can also be worn without interfering with diaper changes and is easily cleaned. For the infant with an unrepaired my-

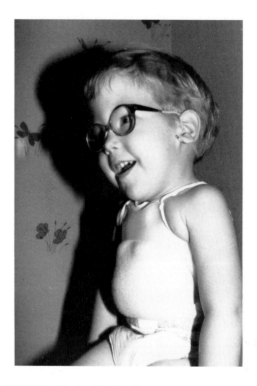

FIGURE 7. Bivalved TLSO with anterior thoracic window.

elomeningocele, the use of a custom molded orthoplast bubble secured with straps around the waist, chest, and shoulders may be necessary to protect the fragile tissues at the site of the defect.[9] After stable concentric reduction of the hips has been accomplished, the prevention of range of motion contractures at the hip, knee, and ankle must be addressed.

If passive range of motion exercise is not sufficient to maintain range of motion in the growing infant, a Newington Positional Orthosis can be useful. Constructed of Vitrathene (a flexible thermoplastic), this posterior half shell covers the feet, legs, and back of the infant holding the legs in extension, abduction, and slight internal rotation to provide concentric reduction of the hips. This orthosis is used during months 3 through 8 and is worn at nighttime and naps. As the infant nears 6 months of age, the addition of hip joints is possible to assist the infant with sitting.[10]

The presence of foot deformities at birth often requires the use of a plastic ankle foot orthosis to assist the orthopedist in maintaining position gained with surgery and in preventing contractures due to muscle imbalance. As equino-varus deformities account for 46% of the foot problems encountered in my-elomeningocele the accurate control of the subtalar joint is essential.[8]

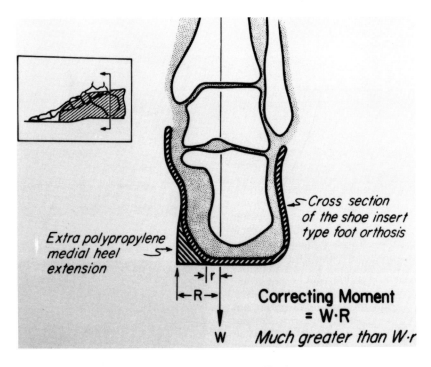

Extra polypropylene medial heel extension

Cross section of the shoe insert type foot orthosis

Correcting Moment
= W·R
Much greater than W·r

FIGURE 8. Gillette heel modification.

The design techniques as described by Carlson and Berglund are quite useful when dealing with the unstable subtalar joint.[11] These authors stress the importance of the accurate and intimate support of the anatomy of the foot and describe mold modifications that enhance calcaneal stability. Complementing this is the use of the Gillette polypropylene medial heel extension to increase the stability of the orthosis inside of the shoe when standing and ambulation are indicated (Figure 8). As the plastic ankle foot orthosis is commonly worn day and night, it is essential that the caregiver be instructed on proper skin care with frequent skin examinations.

Initially the child is weaned into the orthosis until full-time wearing can be tolerated. A well-constructed total contact ankle foot orthosis in the hands of well-informed parents is virtually trouble-free.

At 6 months, the normal infant is attempting to sit and develop further head control. If this is not possible with the myelomeningocele patient due to a thoracic or high lumbar lesion level, a thoracolumbarsacral orthosis (TLSO) is useful in providing trunk stability and subsequently allows the infant to develop further head and neck control. The TLSO is fabricated from 1/8-in. polypropylene copolymer and is bivalved with a window at the chest anteriorly to accommodate chest expansion. Careful attention is needed in the construc-

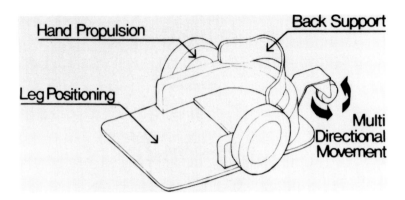

FIGURE 9. Caster cart.

tion of this orthosis to prevent irritation at the site of the myelomeningocele. Foam lining is contraindicated as it is susceptible to contamination by feces and urine[8] (Figure 7).

During months 8 to 12, the normal infant is crawling and developing the head, neck, and torso balance preparatory to standing and walking. The reciprocal movements associated with crawling as well as the increased opportunities to explore their environment are of significant importance to the growth and development of the myelomeningocele patient.

Crawling can be promoted through the use of a variety of adaptive aids that allow the infant to pull himself across the floor with his hands. The Newington "Bug", the "Crawligator" (as described by Carroll in 1974), and the Ontario Crippled Children's Centre caster cart are among a few of the devices designed to assist the infant with early mobility (Figure 9). Crawling without this device should be discouraged as these children are susceptible to decubitus ulcers over the anesthetic portions of their legs.[10]

By the time the child is 12 to 15 months of age, a daily standing program should be initiated. Regular standing will improve renal draining and is thought to promote bone mineralization, although studies supporting this belief have yet to be accomplished. The psychosocial benefits of standing and independent ambulation are significant in that they allow the child to interact with their peer group at eye level and foster a feeling of independence.

A fixed stander with immobile knee and hips joints may be used initially and are relatively inexpensive (Figure 10). As the child approaches preschool age, a parapodium orthosis is desirable as it allows automatic locking and manual unlocking of the knees and hips for seated activities (Figure 11). These devices are used with a parallel rolling walker with some children progressing to Canadian forearm crutches. The addition of a swivel walker attachment enhances the child's mobility by increasing the efficiency of ambulation (Figure 12). During ambulation with a swivel walker attachment, the child will demonstrate a reciprocal lateral trunk shift gait.[19,23] As the child reaches 18 to 24

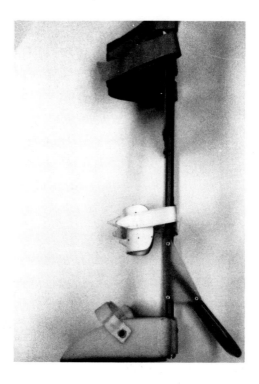

FIGURE 10. Stander.

months of age, decisions regarding his future ambulatory status will come under consideration. Following are some of the factors that are significant in determining the degree to which a child will succeed in developing ambulation skills.

1. The neurosegmental level of the paraplegia
2. The degree of lower extremity deformity
3. The energy demands of ambulation
4. The efficiency and weight of the orthotic system
5. The extent of the spinal deformity
6. Obesity
7. The age and when first braced
8. The child's motivation
9. The extent and quality of the parental involvement in the rehabilitation program
10. The child's cognitive development
11. Upper extremity function

The extent with which these variables combine to affect the ambulatory

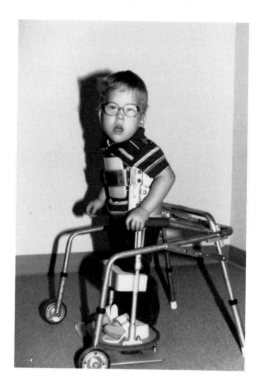

FIGURE 11.   Parapodium.

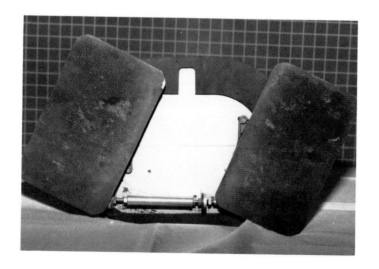

FIGURE 12.   Orlau swivel attachment.

status of the child is a subject that is of considerable interest to the clinic team. The neurosegmental level is considered to be a significant factor in determining ambulation potential.

Stillwell[17] reports on 50 patients from 15 to 31 years of age and compares lesion level to community level ambulation status as follows: sacral, 100%; low lumbar, 95%; high lumbar, 30%; thoracic, 33%.

Hoffer[27] gives us these statistics for a younger population of 56 patients: sacral, 100%; low lumbar, 38%; high lumbar, 31%; thoracic, 0%.

According to Asher[13] patients with fifth lumbar and sacral neurosegmental level paralysis are typically strong community level ambulators.

Patients with fourth lumbar level paraplegia were functional household and community ambulators and the significant variables affecting ambulatory status are (listed in order of importance) the age when first braced and stood, spinal deformity, pelvic obliquity, hip deformity, and knee-foot-ankle deformity. The author states that this neurosegmental level has the most to gain in terms of ambulatory status with proper musculoskeletal care.

Patients with third lumbar neurosegmental level paraplegia were mostly nonfunctional ambulators with the significant variable being hip deformity. Of the third lumbar patients without hip dislocation, 42% were functional ambulators.

Ambulatory status for the first and second lumbar neurosegmental level was most often dependent on obesity and age. The thoracic level paraplegic was most adversely affected by age and knee-foot-ankle deformities. This author emphasizes the importance of controlling obesity and musculoskeletal deformity and suggests that energy expenditure is related to a significant degree with ambulatory status although energy studies were not part of his study.

Stillwell reports fixed flexion deformity at the hip, pelvic obliquity, and scoliosis as significant to the ambulation status of the high lumbar and thoracic neurosegmental level patient.[17]

The L4 sacral neurosegmental level patient has the greatest potential for functional community ambulation. The L3 neurosegmental level is capable of community ambulator status but will tend to be nonfunctional if compromised by pelvic asymmetry, scoliosis, and lower extremity range of motion pathology. The L2, L1, and thoracic neurosegmental level has the potential for functional household and limited community ambulation but may be nonfunctional if compromised by obesity, physical apathy, and lower extremity and spinal malalignment pathologies.

The orthotic management of the L5-sacral neurosegmental typically requires the use of the plastic ankle foot orthosis (AFO). The exception to this is the low sacral neurosegmental level where the use of a plastic foot orthosis may be necessary if pronation (eversion) deformities are present.

Careful attention is required to the selection of the appropriate ankle angulation when designing the plastic AFO. Placing the orthosis in either dorsi- or planterflexion will channel floor reaction forces to the weak or unstable

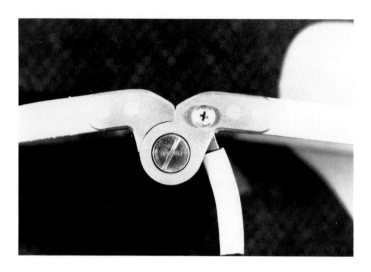

FIGURE 13.   Posterior offset knee joint on KAFO.

knee. The AFO that is fabricated with a rigid ankle section and set in 2 to 5° of planterflexion will generate extensions forces at the knee to supplement weak quadriceps. The extension force is generated over the pretibial muscula- ture when treating the child and the patellar tendon when treating the adult.

When hyperextension due to weak hamstring musculature is present, the use of 2 to 7° of dorsiflexion in the AFO will generate a flexion moment at heel strike and load the quadriceps through stance. When using floor reaction forces in this manner strong quadriceps are necessary.

When inversion-eversion instability is present at the ankle, the use of a lateral or medial extension proximal to the malleolus, in conjunction with the Carlson-Berglund modifications presented previously, will provide additional control. The young child presenting with this lesion level will often require the initial use of a plastic KAFO to protect the ligament structure of the knee. This orthosis is fabricated with a posterior offset knee joint and requires no knee locking mechanism. The use of the posterior offset knee joint offers a bi- omechanical advantage toward extension providing additional stability for the child with fair quadriceps strength (Figure 13). The transition into plastic AFOs is made when concerns over knee stability lessen due to growth.

The L-4 neurosegmental level will occasionally require the initial use of plastic HKAFOs to assist in the prevention of hip flexion contractures and to help control excessive lordosis during stance phase. The presence of knee flexion and hip abduction of grade 3 or better will provide additional pelvic stability and allow the child to transition into bilateral plastic KAFOs.[15,25]

The L-3 through thoracic neurosegmental level provides the clinic team with significant challenges. According to Asher,[13] the most frequent transition in ambulatory status with this group is downward. The child, properly managed, with a level pelvis and no significant lower extremity deformities may still find the energy demands of ambulation, when approaching adulthood, far too great and may eventually choose the wheelchair as the primary form of mobility. This does not, however, negate the numerous physiological and developmental benefits of standing accrued during childhood.

Energy studies comparing swing through ambulation using conventional metal HKAFO systems and the energy demands of wheelchair use illustrate this downward progression in ambulatory status as a function of age, obesity, and physical apathy.[12] As the energy demands of ambulation become too great with age, the natural sequelae of obesity and physical apathy are sure to follow.

The emphasis of modern orthotic care is to reduce these energy demands and provide the high lumbar and thoracic lesion level patient a more attractive alternative to the exclusive use of the wheelchair for mobility. The use of plastics has reduced the weight of the HKAOF system by as much as 50% when compared to conventional metal systems. The use of rigid plastic ankle sections instead of the metal caliper allows the patient to wear a more fashionable footwear with improved cosmesis. Plastic HKAFO systems with locked hips and knees require the patient to use a swing-through gait pattern for ambulation. The energy inefficiency of this type of gait pattern, even with a lighter orthosis, continues to be a significant bar to long-term functional ambulation.[16,22]

The development of the reciprocation gait orthosis (RGO) as described by Motlock and further developed by Douglas provides us with some answers to this difficult problem.[20,28] The function of this orthosis allows the child to ambulate with a four-point reciprocal gait pattern, reducing the need for the child's upper extremities to carry significant portions of the body weight through swing phase by providing the child with a reciprocal stance phase during gait.

The RGO is a dual cable-controlled hip mechanism that utilizes the hip flexion of one extremity to provide reciprocal hip extension to the opposite extremity. The upper extremities are used primarily for balance and, with the absence of hip flexors in the thoracic lesion level, to propel the child forward through the gait cycle (Figure 14).

Contraindications for this device are hip and knee flexion contractures greater than 10°, unilateral hip dislocation, pelvic asymmetry, and significant spinal curvatures.

According to energy studies conducted by Flandry at Louisiana State University Medical Center, the energy expenditure for ambulation with the RGO approximates that found in wheelchair use.[14]

Due to the complex nature of this device, careful consideration by a multidisciplinary team that is familiar with the candidate's background is essential. The extensive physical therapy prior to and after fabrication of the orthosis requires a considerable time commitment on the part of the patient and family.

After the orthosis has been successfully fit and the patient trained in its use,

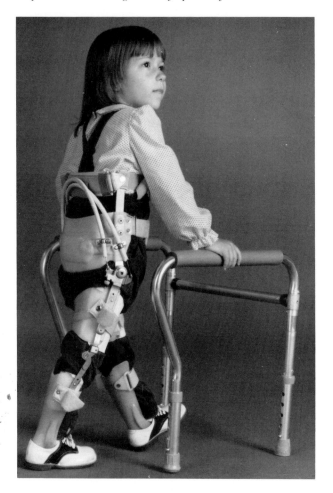

FIGURE 14.   RGO dual cable hip control mechanism.

periodic adjustments to accommodate for growth will be necessary at 3-month intervals.[26]

The RGO represents a significant advance in energy-efficient orthotics for the high lumbar and thoracic level myelomeningocele patient. Ultimately, the transition into this device and the child's subsequent success with it are dependent to a large extent on the quality of the orthopedic and orthotic care the child receives during his first 2 years of life.

III. SEATING THE MYELOMENINGOCELE PATIENT WITH THE GILLETTE SITTING SUPPORT ORTHOSIS

It is beyond the scope of this chapter to present the multitude of devices currently available to seat the multiply handicapped child and young adult. The

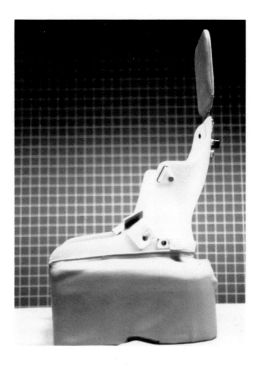

FIGURE 15. Gillette sitting support orthosis.

majority of children with myelomeningocele can be seated effectively with fairly simple seating systems that assist in positioning the lower extremities and provide cushioning to the pelvis and buttocks. A small minority of these children present considerable challenges to the clinic team due to a combination of deformities that substantially increase their risk for the development of pressure decubitus.[21] According to Drummond,[24] the high neurosegmental level nonambulating myelomeningocele patient with pelvic obliquity, scoliosis, hypolordosis is at risk for the development of pressure decubitus. The combination of these risk factors leads to abnormal pressure distribution on and about the ischium and sacrococcygeal areas. Drummond demonstrates that a shift of weight greater than 30% under one ischium, 11% under the sacrococcygeal area or greater than 55% of the total weight distributed to these three areas increases the likelihood of pressure decubitus.

It has been the experience of our office that the Gillette Sitting Support Orthosis (SSO) is of use in seating this type of patient. The SSO is a plastic copolymer polypropylene posterior shell fabricated from an impression taken of the patient in the prone position with hips and knees in flexion (Figure 15). Careful attention is directed at placing reliefs over pressure intolerant tissues and directing this pressure to adjacent pressure tolerant tissues.[29]

Inherent in the design of this orthosis is the ability to stabilize the pelvis in such a manner as to ensure accurate and consistent approximation of the bony prominences over the reliefs necessary to protect them. This is especially advantageous in the patient with a kypholordotic spine deformity. In addition, this device allows the accurate control of hip and knee flexion angles that are so essential to the optimization of head and torso balance.

The materials used to fabricate this orthosis are appropriate for the incontinent patient and the portability of this device provides for the seating needs of the patient away from the wheelchair.

IV. CONCLUSION

The challenges of providing orthotic care for the child with myelomeningocele are best answered by the cooperative efforts of the multidisciplinary clinic team. The emphasis of early orthotic care is to assist the orthopedist in correcting and maintaining musculoskeletal alignment and to assist the child in attaining the usual developmental milestones of sitting, crawling, standing and walking.

The transition from standing to walking is dependent on a number of factors that influence the functional status the child may eventually achieve. Advances in orthotic fabrication technology in recent years have enhanced the functional potential of these individuals by providing them with lightweight orthotic devices that minimize the energy demands placed on the patient during ambulation.

It is our hope that these advances ultimately provide these patients with enhanced functional capabilities and a higher quality of life.

REFERENCES

1. **Brunt, D.,** Predictive factors of perceptual motor ability in children with meningomyelocele, *Am. Correct. Ther. J.*, 35(2), 42, 1981.
2. **Hayden, P. W.,** Adolescents with myelodysplasia: impact of physical disability on emotional maturation, *Pediatrics*, 64(1), 53, 1988.
3. **Hunt, G. M.,** Factors relating to intelligence in treated cases of spina bifida cystica, *Am. J. Disab. Child*, 130, 823, 1976.
4. **Asher, M.,** The Myelomeningocele patient. A multidisciplinary approach to care, *J. Kans. Med. Soc.*, 80(7), 403, 1979.
5. **Scarff, T.,** Myelomeningocele: a review and update, *Rehabil. Lit.*, 42(5–6), 143, 1981.
6. **Soare, P.,** Intellectual and perceptual-motor characteristics of treated myelomeningocele children, *Am. J. Disab. Child*, 131, 199, 1977.
7. **Feldman, W.,** A parent training program for the child with spina bifida, *Spina Bifida Ther.*, 4(2), 77, 1982.
8. **Bunch, W.,** Myelomeningocele, *Pediatr. Orthoped.*, 1986, 1(2), 397, 1986.
9. **Passo, S. D.,** Positioning infants with myelomeningocele, *Am. J. Nurs.*, 74(9), 1658, 1974.

10. **Drennan, J. C.,** Orthotic management of the myelomeningocele spine, *Dev. Med. Child Neurol.,* 18(Suppl. 37), 97, 1976.

11. **Carlson, J. M.,** An effective orthotic design for controlling the unstable subtalar joint, *Orthotic. Prosth.,* 33(1), 33, 1979.

12. **Evans, E. P.,** Energy expenditure and movement among children with myelomeningocele, *Spina Bifida Ther.,* 4(2), 43, 1989.

13. **Asher, M.,** Factors affecting the ambulatory status of patients with spina bifida cystica, *J. Bone Jt. Surg.,* 65A(3), 350, 1983.

14. **Flandry, F.,** Functional ambulation in myelodysplasia: the effect of orthotic selection on physical and physiologic performance, *J. Pediatr. Orthoped.,* 6(6), 661, 1986.

15. **Glancy, C. O.,** A dynamic orthotic system for young myelomeningoceles, *Orthotic. Prosth.,* 30(4), 3, 1976.

16. **Rose, G. K.,** Clinical evaluation of spina bifida patients using hip guidance orthosis, *Dev. Med. Child Neurol.,* 23, 30, 1981.

17. **Stillwell, A.,** Walking ability in mature patients with spina bifida, *J. Pediatr. Orthoped.,* 3(2), 184, 1983.

18. **Carroll, N. C.,** Assessment and management of the lower extremity in myelodysplasia, *Orthoped. Clin. N. Am.,* 14(4), 709, 1987.

19. **Lough, L. K.,** Ambulation of children with myelomeningocele: parapodium versus parapodium with the Orlau swivel modification, *Dev. Med. Child Neurol.,* 28(4), 661, 1986.

20. **Yngve, D. A.,** The reciprocating gait orthosis in myelomeningocele, *J. Pediatr. Orthoped.,* 4(3), 304, 1984.

21. **Okamoto, G. A.,** Skin breakdown in patients with myelomeningocele, *Arch. Phys. Med. Rehabil.,* 64(1), 20, 1983.

22. **Stallard, J.,** Assessment of orthosis by means of speed and heart rate, *J. Med. Eng. Technol.,* 2(1), 22, 1978.

23. **Griffiths, J. C.,** Clinical applications of the paraplegic swivel walker, *J. Biomed. Eng.,* 2(4), 250, 1980.

24. **Drummond, D.,** Relationship of spine deformity and pelvic obliquity on sitting pressure distributions and decubitus ulceration, *J. Pediatr. Orthoped.,* 5(4), 396, 1985.

25. **Glancy, J.,** Dynamics and the L3 through L5 myelomeningocele child, *Clin. Prosthet. Orthotics,* 8(4), 15, 1984.

26. **Supan, T. J.,** Orthotic management program for the myelodysplastic child, *Clin. Prosthet. Orthotics,* 8(4), 12, 1984.

27. **Hoffer, M. M.,** Functional ambulation in patients with myelomeningocele, *J. Bone Jt. Surg.,* 55, 137, 1973.

28. **Douglas, R.,** The LSU reciprocation-gait orthosis, *Orthopedics,* 6, 834, 1983.

29. **Carlson, J.,** Seating for children and young adults with cerebral palsy, *Clin. Orthotic. Prosthet.,* 10(4), 137, 1986.

Chapter 8

UROLOGIC MANAGEMENT OF SPINA BIFIDA

Robert B. Bailey

TABLE OF CONTENTS

Spina bifida patients have a wide variety of urological problems. In the past, the frequent cause of death in these patients was secondary to urological complications. Over the last 15 years, the urologic management of spina bifida has changed dramatically, especially with the introduction of clean intermittent catheterization. However, over 95% of children will have urinary incontinence if untreated.[1] The urological care of children with spina bifida should begin in the neonatal period with urological consultation being mandatory during the initial hospitalization. This chapter provides for the personnel involved in the care of patients with spina bifida an understanding of the underlying problem and a rational plan for evaluation and subsequent management.

I. NORMAL LOWER URINARY TRACT

A. Anatomy

The normal bladder wall is composed of three distinct layers of muscle fibers. These include the inner longitudinal, middle circular, and outer longitudinal layers. The bladder is divided into (1) the fundus, which comprises most of the bladder wall and determines the capacity of the bladder; (2) the trigone, into which the ureters empty; and (3) the bladder neck, which functions as the involuntary internal sphincter. The bladder empties into the urethra which passes through the urogenital diaphragm which is the area where the external sphincter lies. The external sphincter is comprised of the striated muscles of the pelvic floor and is under voluntary control (Figure 1).

B. Nerve Supply

The nerve supply to the bladder and external sphincter comprises a group of nerves from the sympathetic, parasympathetic, and somatic nerve groups.

Motor innervation to the muscles of the fundus of the bladder arise from the parasympathetic nerves at the S-2, S-3, and S-4 level which control bladder

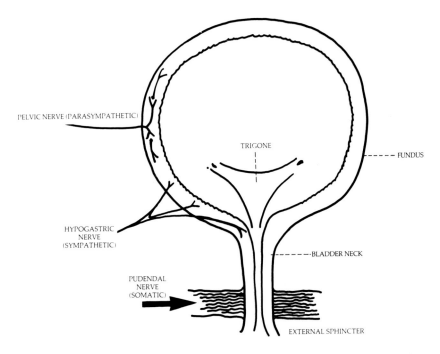

FIGURE 1. Diagram depicting the anatomy of the bladder with its motor and sensory innervation.

contraction. Sympathetic nerves from the thoracolumbar outflow tract from T-11 through L-2 innervate the bladder neck area and result in internal sphincter control. The motor nerves to the external sphincter arise from the pudendal nerve coming from S-2, S-3, and S-4. The afferent sensory nerves from the area of the bladder neck and trigone travel through the sympathetic trunk to T-11, T-12, L-1, and L-2.

C. Bladder Physiology

Normal bladder physiology allows for the storage of urine at low pressures with the subsequent emptying of the bladder through contraction of the detrusor muscle in coordination with relaxation of both the internal and external sphincters. The phenomenon of micturition is under voluntary control in the normal situation. A coordinated voiding reflex is important in maintaining low intravesical pressures in order to prevent the development of upper urinary tract dilation which develops secondary to an increased backpressure effect (Figure 2A).

II. LOWER URINARY TRACT IN SPINA BIFIDA

A. Abnormal Bladder Physiology

The neuropathic bladder is the underlying problem that results in the urologic complications of spina bifida. Spina bifida patients have a combination of

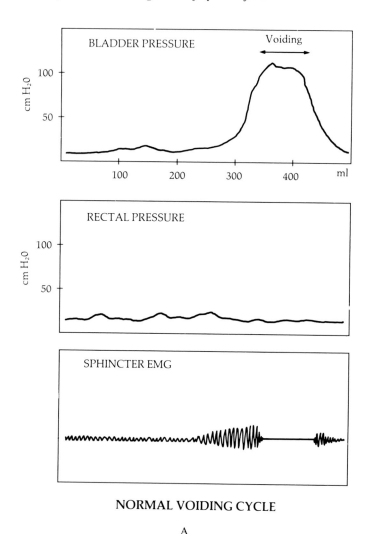

NORMAL VOIDING CYCLE

A

FIGURE 2. (A) Urodynamic study of a normal voiding cycle. Note the decreased EMG signal during voiding. (B) Urodynamic study revealing bladder sphincter dyssynergia. Note the increased EMG signal during voiding.

an upper and a lower motor neuron type of neurogenic bladder dysfunction that is the result of the complex neurological deficit created by the myelomeningocele. The type of neurogenic bladder in an individual patient is not predictable by the level of the bony defect in most cases but is determined by the degree of malformation of the spinal cord and nerve roots which is variable. However, there are different basic types of neurogenic bladders that allow the urologist to group patients into separate categories allowing for a rational treatment plan.

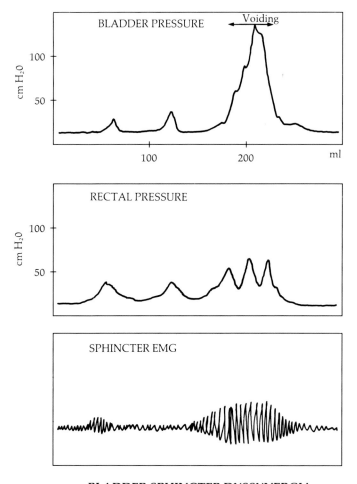

BLADDER SPHINCTER DYSSYNERGIA

FIGURE 2B.

B. Types of Neurogenic Bladders in Spina Bifida
1. Hypertonic Bladder

The hypertonic bladder or spastic bladder is one in which the voiding reflex arc is intact but is essentially uninhibited. These bladders develop high intravesical pressures resulting in secondary back pressure to the upper urinary tract. There is a lack of efficient regulation from higher brain centers resulting in the spastic behavior. The hypertonic bladder will develop a thickened muscular wall with subsequent development of cellules and saccules of the bladder wall. These features are readily identifiable on X-ray examination. Over time, hypertonic bladders tend to become small in capacity.

2. Hypotonic Bladder

The hypotonic or flaccid bladder is secondary to disruption of the sacral cord segments that result in a flaccid paralysis of the bladder. This type of bladder has low resting pressures and detrusor contractions are extremely weak or absent. Dilation of the upper urinary tract results from chronic overdistension of the bladder. X-ray examination of a flaccid bladder usually reveals a thin, smooth-walled bladder.

C. Sphincteric Dysfunction

Urinary continence is determined by the relationship of bladder function in combination with sphincteric function. There are many different combinations of bladder dysfunction and sphincteric difficulties that result in urinary incontinence. In order to have urinary incontinence, either the intravesical pressure generated from a bladder contraction is higher than normally adequate outflow resistance, or the outflow resistance is inadequate regardless of bladder pressure. However, there is another form of voiding dysfunction that is called bladder-sphincter dyssynergia, which occurs when there is an uncoordinated voiding reflex. As the bladder contracts, the external or internal sphincters remain contracted rather than relaxing, resulting in increased intravesical pressure and subsequent upper urinary tract dilation (Figure 2B).

III. UPPER URINARY TRACT ANATOMY IN SPINA BIFIDA

Upper urinary tract anomalies are relatively common in spina bifida. Roberts found that 18% of patients with myelomeningocele at autopsy had anomalies of the urinary tract exclusive of hydroureter or hydronephrosis that could have been secondary to the underlying neurogenic bladder.[2] Horseshoe kidney was the most common abnormality with crossed renal ectopia and renal agenesis not uncommon. Recently, Fernback and Davis suggested that many instances of horseshoe kidney are actually pseudohorseshoe kidney which are secondary to the thoracolumbar Gibbis deformity in patients with thoracolumbar myelomeningocoele.[3]

IV. COMPLICATIONS OF NEUROGENIC BLADDERS

The major complications of the neurogenic bladder include urinary incontinence, urinary tract infection, and hydronephrosis which includes vesicoureteral reflux.

A. Urinary Incontinence

If left untreated, 95% of children with myelomeningocele will have urinary incontinence.[1] The urinary incontinence is secondary to the underlying neurogenic bladder. It is helpful to distinguish between those patients whose bladders fail to store urine as compared to those patients whose bladders are not able to empty urine. Inability to store urine may be secondary to a hypertonic bladder, a small capacity bladder, or a lower urinary tract that has inadequate outlet resistance. Urinary incontinence may arise from one or a combination of all three of these factors. The goal when treating incontinence in patients with spina bifida is to determine which one of these factors or combination of factors is present and develop the appropriate treatment plan. The majority of children with spina bifida can achieve social continence through the use of clean intermittent catheterization (CIC) in combination with either pharmacological agents, various types of bladder surgery, or placement of an artificial urinary sphincter.

B. Urinary Tract Infection

Urinary tract infection is common in patients with a neurogenic bladder. Infection used to be a common cause of mortality in patients with spina bifida. In the past, the common use of indwelling urinary catheters led to a high incidence of infection. Although chronic bacilluria is common with CIC, the morbidity is low in the absence of vesicoureteral reflux. Kass et al. found bacteriuria in 56% of 255 children on CIC.[4] Febrile urinary tract infections occurred in only 3% of patients without vesicoureteral reflux. However, 37% of the patients with reflux developed febrile urinary tract infections emphasizing the significant morbidity of CIC in the presence of vesicoureteral reflux.

C. Hydronephrosis

The hydronephrosis exclusive of congenital obstructive uropathies that develops in patients with spina bifida is caused in most cases by two phenomena that are interrelated, the neurogenic bladder and vesicoureteral reflux. As a result of the bladder hypertonicity present in the neurogenic bladder, there is increased intravesical pressure that results in the development of upper urinary tract dilation. McGuire and co-workers have shown with their urodynamic testing in spina bifida patients that of those patients whose intravesical pressure at the time of urethral leakage of urine was 40 cm of water or greater, 81% showed evidence of upper urinary tract dilation on excretory urography.[5]

The other complication of the neurogenic bladder that results in hydronephrosis is the development of vesicoureteral reflux. In a neurogenic bladder, this is due to decompensation of the ureterovesical junction which is secondary to a combination of both high intravesical pressure and the abnormal bladder wall muscle; consequently, there is reflux of urine back into the upper urinary tract. McGuire and co-workers found that in patients whose urethral leakage pressure was 40 cm of water or greater, 68% showed evidence of vesicoureteral reflux.[5]

Kaplan and co-workers found an incidence of hydronephrosis in 23% of newborns with myelodysplasia.[6] However, they showed that in some patients, the hydronephrosis was transient and limited to the acute period after neurosurgical closure of the back. Treatment of the hydronephrosis secondary to neurovesical dysfunction in the newborn involves starting CIC or the creation of a cutaneous vesicostomy. Although it originally had been felt that CIC could not be performed on newborn males, it has been shown that a catheterization program is feasible.[7] If a family is unable to perform catheterization, then a cutaneous vesicostomy is indicated. Enrile and Crooks looked at the effect on upper tract dilation in response to intermittent catheterization.[8] They detected an improvement in the dilation in 38% of patients and there was stabilization in 46% but a progression of upper tract deterioration in 16%.

D. Calculi

Urinary calculi in patients with spina bifida are usually due to an infectious etiology. These stones usually consist of struvite and are associated with urea splitting organisms such as proteus. Stone treatment in spina bifida patients is no different than in the general urological population. Treatment should include an attempt to eradicate the potential for recurrence by trying to eliminate urinary tract infection in susceptible patients.

V. UROLOGIC EVALUATION IN SPINA BIFIDA

The urological evaluation of the patient with spina bifida should begin early in the neonatal period. While the neurosurgical problem is the primary concern initially, the baby should be promptly evaluated by the pediatric urologist as soon as possible after back closure. It is important at that point to document urinary tract anatomy and detect any underlying abnormalities, such as hydronephrosis, which would be suggestive of early deterioration of the urinary tract. Recently, it has been shown that early detection of neurovesical dysfunction can prevent the development of early upper urinary tract deterioration by instituting aggressive bladder management programs early in the newborn period.[9]

A. Upper Urinary Tract Evaluation

The initial urological imaging study obtained in the newborn period should be a renal and pelvic ultrasound. The ultrasound examination is an excellent modality for screening the urinary tract for hydronephrosis, as well as documenting renal anatomy and the presence of two kidneys (Figure 3). Duplicated systems can also be diagnosed using renal ultrasonography. While utilizing no radiation, it is an excellent noninvasive test. Gaum and co-workers discovered an abnormal upper urinary tract in 19% of a group of 68 neonates with spina bifida.[10]

The ultrasound examination does not provide information about kidney function. When the ultrasound examination demonstrates hydronephrosis or ureterectasis and the voiding cystourethrogram shows no reflux, further investigation with an upper urinary tract function test is indicated. Depending on the

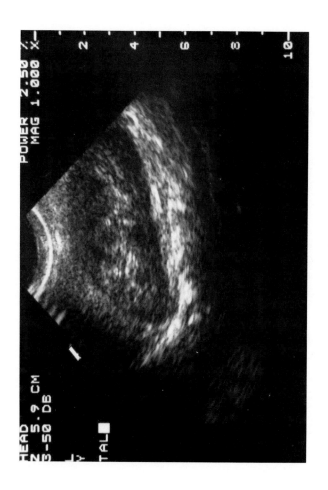

A

FIGURE 3. (A) Normal renal ultrasound and (B) abnormal renal ultrasound showing hydronephrosis.

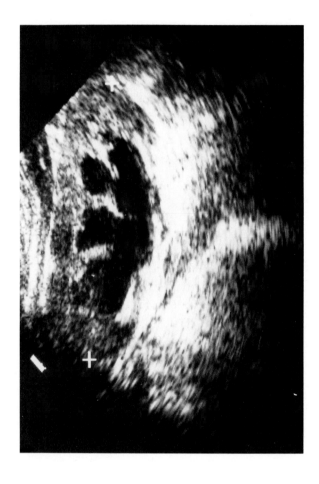

FIGURE 3B.

ultrasound findings, the next imaging test would be either an intravenous pyelogram (IVP) or a nuclear renal scan. The IVP is an X-ray study where dye is injected intravenously with the kidneys excreting the dye, thereby providing visualization or urinary tract anatomy, including the renal parenchyma, renal pelvis, and ureters. However, it is less optimal in visualizing bladder anatomy. Although one can infer from the IVP the degree of obstruction, it is best used to isolate the level of obstruction and display the anatomy.

The nuclear renal scan with DTPA is used for evaluating renal function and the degree of urinary tract obstruction but is suboptimal in outlining urinary tract anatomy. However, in many cases of obstructive uropathy, fine detail of the anatomy is not required but a relatively precise determination of the degree of obstruction is desired. The DTPA scan, through the use of computer analysis, can provide washout times for the excretion of the radionucleotide. From experience it has been determined which washout times are acceptable and which are indicative of significant urinary tract obstruction.

Both the IVP and DTPA renal scan can be difficult to interpret in the early neonatal period. Therefore, these tests should be delayed until at least 1 to 2 weeks of life is possible. In cases where it cannot be determined whether a system is obstructed after IVP or renal scan, a Whittaker test is sometimes utilized.[11] The Whittaker test involves placing a precutaneous nephrostomy tube while simultaneously placing a bladder catheter. The renal pelvis pressure and bladder pressure are measured simultaneously as normal saline is instilled through the nephrostomy tube into the kidney. A differential of <15 cm of water pressure between bladder and renal pelvis indicates a significant obstruction.

B. Lower Urinary Tract Evaluation

The voiding cystourethrogram (VCUG) is an excellent examination for evaluating lower urinary tract anatomy. It also provides indirect information about lower urinary tract function. A VCUG is performed by placing a urinary catheter in the bladder and instilling radiopaque dye. As the bladder is filled with dye, the bladder outline is demonstrated. The normal bladder shows a smooth outline, while the abnormal, neurogenic bladder seen in children with spina bifida will demonstrate an irregular outline with diverticula in some cases. Vesicoureteral reflux may be witnessed with bladder filling (Figure 4). The catheter is then removed and spontaneous voiding, if possible, is visualized. The degree of vesicoureteral reflux can be graded and the degree of bladder emptying can be assessed with a recording of the postvoid residual.

Gaum and co-workers have shown the necessity of obtaining a VCUG in the neonatal period.[10] They found an abnormal VCUG in 69% of neonates with normal upper tract examinations. Of patients with an abnormal upper tract examination, 92% had an abnormal VCUG that included those patients with vesicoureteral reflux, diverticulum formation, and bladder wall irregularity of a mild or marked degree. Very small capacity bladders, as well as those

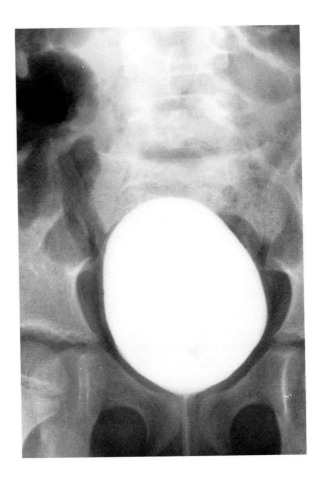

A

FIGURE 4. (A) Normal cystogram revealing smooth-walled bladder
and (B) abnormal cystogram revealing trabeculated bladder and severe
bilateral vesicoureteral reflux.

displaying the Christmas tree type of pattern were considered abnormal.
Vesicoureteral reflux was found in 15% of patients with normal upper urinary
tracts, while 23% of patients with abnormal upper tracts demonstrated vesicoureteral reflux. These data illustrate that relying solely on an ultrasound
study of the upper tracts will lead to an underdiagnosis of patients with
abnormal urinary tracts.

C. Urodynamic Studies

Urodynamic testing has been an invaluable addition to the examinations
used for evaluating children with spina bifida. Urodynamic testing involves the

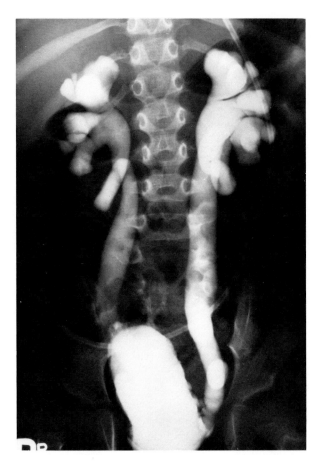

FIGURE 4B.

placement of a triple lumen urinary catheter that allows simultaneous measurement of bladder and urethral pressures. A rectal pressure monitor is also placed as well as an EMG electrode, either on the surface of the perineal skin or as a needle electrode into the striated muscle of the external sphincter. With filling of the bladder through the triple lumen catheter, the different pressures are recorded with bladder contraction allowing one to evaluate the efficiency and coordination of micturition. Only with urodynamic testing can bladder sphincter dyssynergia be documented (Figures 2A and B).

In the past, urodynamic evaluation of patients with spina bifida was not performed until the children were older and had shown evidence of urinary tract deterioration. Recently, it has been shown that urodynamic evaluation can be undertaken in the newborn period with relative ease. Bauer and co-workers performed urodynamic evaluations on 36 infants with myelodysplasia.[9] Of the infants, 50% showed evidence of bladder sphincter dyssynergia while 25% had coordinated activity of the external sphincter with 25% showing no activity of the external sphincter.

Only 3 of 18 infants with bladder sphincter dyssynergia had evidence of hydronephrosis on their initial upper tract imaging study, but 72% of the patients with bladder sphincter dyssynergia were eventually found to have decompensation of the urinary tract as evidenced by the development of severe hydroureteronephrosis, massive reflux, or an enlarged bladder with a large postvoiding volume of urine. This compared to the development of upper tract deterioration in 22% of patients without bladder sphincter dyssynergia and 11% of those with no activity of the external sphincter.[9]

McGuire and co-workers demonstrated the relationship between the urethral closure pressure and intravesical pressure at the time of urethral leakage in a group of patients with myelodysplasia.[5] In 20 patients whose intravesical pressure at the time of urethral leakage was 40 cm of water or less, none had vesicoureteral reflux and two showed evidence of ureteral dilation on excretory urography. In the 22 patients whose intravesical pressure at the time of urethral leakage was 40 cm of water or greater, 68% showed vesicoureteral reflux and 81% showed ureteral dilation on excretory urography. Sidi et al. performed a prospective study looking at the value of urodynamic testing of neonates with myelodysplasia.[12] They found that in patients with low pressure bladders and coordinated bladder and sphincter activity, those with normal radiographic findings initially remained normal whereas in those with initially abnormal radiographic findings, 67% reversed to normal without treatment, 17% remained stable, and 17% had deterioration.

The use of urodynamic testing in the newborn period allows for the identification of those patients who are at greatest risk for developing upper urinary tract deterioration and require intermittent catheterization or vesicostomy starting in the newborn period.

VI. UROLOGIC MANAGEMENT OF SPINA BIFIDA

A. Timing of Urologic Evaluation

The urological management of the patient with spina bifida should begin early in the neonatal period. As discussed previously, an upper tract imaging study and VCUG should be obtained, while the benefit of urodynamic testing in the neonatal period has also been outlined. If urodynamic testing is not performed, then frequent upper tract imaging studies to detect the presence of upper tract deterioration will be necessary. If the initial imaging studies are abnormal, showing hydroureteronephrosis or vesicoureteral reflux, then treatment should be initiated in the neonatal period with either clean intermittent catheterization or creation of a vesicostomy in addition to anticholinergic medication. It is preferred that urodynamic testing be obtained in order to document the underlying neurovesical dysfunction, while also providing a baseline in order to evaluate the efficacy of the treatment program initiated. In those patients with upper urinary tract deterioration, frequent upper tract imaging studies are needed and should be obtained every 6 months until it is certain that the upper tracts have stabilized. Follow-up urodynamic testing is usually obtained approximately 6 months after initiating a treatment program.

If the initial imaging studies are within normal limits, then urodynamic studies can identify those patients at risk for developing upper urinary tract deterioration. However, if urodynamic studies are not obtained, then a follow-up ultrasound examination should be obtained 3 to 4 months after birth.

Sidi et al. were able to reverse the upper urinary tract changes in 40% of children they found with high pressure bladders and bladder sphincter dyssynergia.[12] They stabilized 40% of the patients while 20% showed signs of deterioration despite anticholinergic medication and CIC or vesicostomy.

Spindel et al. followed 79 newborns with myelodysplasia for up to 6 years with serial imaging studies and urodynamic evaluations beginning in the newborn period.[13] Of the infants, 37% developed changes in external urethral sphincter innervation during the first 3 years of life, 86% demonstrated the change in the 1st year, 10% in the 2nd year, and 4% in the 3rd year. They figured that the risk factor for change was 32% in the 1st year, 6% in the 2nd year, and 2% in the 3rd year.

This report underscores the need for frequent urological evaluations of infants with spina bifida, especially during the first 3 years of life. Not only is it necessary to perform frequent surveillance of those patients with known upper urinary tract deterioration, but it is important to monitor all patients for a changing neurourologic lesion, especially in the 1st year of life. After age 3, evaluations need not be as frequent, but they should be performed at least annually. Of course, those patients with clinical deterioration will need to be followed as frequently as their condition dictates.

B. Intermittent Catheterization

CIC of the bladder through the urethra was introduced in 1972 by Lapides.[14] He demonstrated that a clean, unsterile catheterization technique was possible in those patients who were candidates for intermittent catheterization. Lapides displaced the commonly held belief that intermittent urethral catheterization caused urinary tract infection rather than helping to alleviate infection caused by bladder overdistention. He emphasized that the frequency of catheterization was more important than the sterility of the procedure because preventing bladder overdistention prevented bacterial overgrowth and subsequent urinary tract infection.[14]

The use of CIC revolutionized the treatment of patients with spina bifida. Many patients who were previously thought to be untreatable except with urinary diversion became continent on an intermittent self-catheterization program. In fact, a number of investigators have shown that the upper tract deterioration secondary to the neurogenic bladder in patients with spina bifida will respond favorably to a regimen of intermittent self-catheterization. Enrile and Crooks found that 83% of patients with abnormal upper urinary tracts improved or stabilized on a CIC program.[8] They found no renal deterioration in children on CIC who began with normal upper urinary tracts. Urinary incontinence was improved in 66% of those patients studied.

The majority of patients with spina bifida, after reaching the appropriate age, will tolerate an intermittent self-catheterization program with adequate teaching and psychological support. The patients with the most difficulty are males with normal urethral sensation. In some cases, catheterization has to be done as frequently as every 2 h in order to achieve urinary continence. Such a frequent catheterization schedule can prove to be difficult to maintain on a permanent basis. Some children with severe orthopedic deformities are unable to physically perform self-catheterization due to body habitus, while others have limited manual dexterity precluding self-catheterization and require another individual to perform the catheterization.

In patients with urinary tract deterioration, CIC should be instituted immediately after diagnosis including in the newborn period. Using a small caliber catheter, both male and female newborns have successfully tolerated a catheterization regimen.[7] In newborn patients whose parents are unable to perform catheterization, a cutaneous vesicostomy will be needed as a temporary urinary diversion in order to prevent further deterioration of the upper urinary tract. Kass and associates reported on 42 patients less than 6 years old including small infants on whom an intermittent catheterization program proved successful.[15] The morbidity of intermittent catheterization in children is low but occasionally a male patient will develop a false passage, usually in the bulbous urethra secondary to a traumatic catheterization. This complication may preclude the subsequent use of intermittent catheterization, but it may still be possible with a coudé or curved tip catheter.

The incidence of bacteriuria in patients on intermittent catheterization is quite high. Ehrlich and Brem found only 16% of their patients on intermittent catheterization to have consistently sterile urine.[16] Kass et al. looked at 255 children managed with CIC over a period of 10 years in order to determine the incidence of bacteriuria and upper urinary tract deterioration.[4] Persistent bacteriuria occurred in 56% of the children, but febrile urinary tract infections occurred in only 11% of patients. However, pyelonephritis occurred in more than 60% of patients with high grade vesicoureteral reflux, but the reflux eventually disappeared in up to 50% of cases after initiation of CIC. The morbidity of CIC in those patients without significant vesicoureteral reflux was low with only a 3% incidence of febrile urinary tract infection.

In patients with reflux, close surveillance is required including obtaining frequent urine cultures as well as continuing the patients on prophylactic antibiotics. Since a significant percentage of patients will spontaneously resolve their reflux after initiation of CIC, persistence with the catheterization program is desirable at least temporarily before deciding on surgical correction of the reflux. In those patients on CIC with persistent breakthrough febrile urinary tract infections, changing to a sterile technique will prevent break-through infection in a significant percentage of patients.

The two reasons for initiating an intermittent catheterization program are to achieve urinary continence, and to treat or prevent upper urinary tract deterioration. When using catheterization for treatment of an upper urinary tract problem, the program should begin at the time of diagnosis regardless of the age of the patient. If a catheterization program proves infeasible, then a urinary diversion should be considered. In those patients without upper urinary tract deterioration, a catheterization program should be considered between the ages of 3 and 4 when most children without a neurogenic bladder will have achieved social continence. Many parents, however, elect to defer starting catheterization until the child begins school. Most children by the age of 6 can adequately perform self-catheterization with proper teaching and support.

C. Pharmacological Treatment

The neurogenic bladder in spina bifida responds remarkably well to pharmacological treatment in many cases. Drug therapy in combination with intermittent catheterization can achieve urinary continence in the majority of patients. Pharmacological manipulation is directed toward treating the detrimental physiological actions of the neurogenic bladder.

Detrusor hypertonicity can be counteracted by the use of anticholinergic agents that relax the smooth muscle of the bladder. The most frequently used drugs are oxybutynin and propantheline. Both medications act to decrease intravesical pressure and help increase bladder capacity. These medications may be started empirically when the clinical work-up suggests that they would be beneficial, but it is preferable to perform urodynamic studies prior to initiation of anticholinergic treatment. Many patients with high bladder leak point pressures can effectively reduce their intravesical pressures with anticholinergic medication in combination with intermittent catheterization. Imipramine, which is a tricyclic antidepressant medication, also helps increase bladder capacity and decrease intravesical pressure by causing bladder relaxation.

Decreased outlet resistance caused by an incompetent bladder neck can be effectively treated in some cases by the use of α-sympathomimetic medications. Working on the sympathetic α-receptors of the bladder neck, α-agonists increase outlet resistance and help improve urinary continence. Imipramine also has an effect on the bladder neck resulting in increasing outlet resistance. There is no effective medication that can increase the resistance at the external sphincter level.

Hilwa and Perlmutter looked at adjunctive drug therapy for intermittent catheterization in 39 children with vesical dysfunction in whom the bladder dysfunction was caused by myelodysplasia in the majority of the patients.[17] Of 24 females, 5 were continent day and night without drug therapy on intermittent catheterization, whereas 15 of 16 patients placed on drug therapy in combination with intermittent catheterization became continent. Only 2 of 13 boys were dry on catheterization without drug treatment while 8 of 9 became continent on medication. Bladder capacity increased from an average of 160 to 276 cm^3 after initiation of oxybutynin treatment. These results show the importance of simultaneously treating patients with myelomeningocele on intermittent catheterization with additional pharmacological therapy. Although these results are encouraging, the author's definition of continence included those children who were dry for only 2 h. If one uses the definition of continence as being dry for 3 h during the day, their success rate with this program decreases and identifies those patients who require surgical intervention in order to become socially continent.

D. Surgical Management of Spina Bifida
1. Bladder Augmentation

In those patients with spina bifida who have a small capacity bladder with poor compliance or in those who have severe detrussor hypertonicity unresponsive to catheterization and anticholinergic medicine, the enlargement of the bladder with intestinal segments has proved to be an invaluable modality. Bladder augmentation increases capacity, decreases intravesical pressure, and improves bladder wall compliance. Many patients who have previously undergone supravesical urinary diversion with intestinal segments for intractable incontinence due to their small, noncompliant bladders can be effectively undiverted using bladder augmentation.

Bladder augmentation involves isolating a segment of intestine, either large or small, and after detubularizing the intestinal segment, suturing it to the bladder which has been opened longitudinally (Figure 5). There are two important considerations in this procedure: (1) assuring that the bladder is opened far enough in order to eliminate bladder contractions and prevent an hourglass deformity, and (2) effectively detubularizing the intestinal segment in order to prevent involuntary contractions of the segment that can cause incontinence. Detubularization is accomplished by opening the intestinal segment along its antimesenteric border prior to suturing the segment to the bladder remnant. Although there is some controversy concerning the optimal use of intestinal segments, both ileal and sigmoid segments have been shown to be adequate when effectively detubularized. Caution should be used when considering using the ileal cecal segment in patients with spina bifida since removal of this segment from the intestinal tract may lead to trouble with bowel training secondary to persistent diarrhea. However, many surgeons prefer to use the ilealcecal valve as the method for creating an antirefluxing valve into which the ureters may be placed, thereby effectively reducing vesicoureteral reflux. An alternate and equally successful method is to reimplant the ureters into the bladder remnant, or if not possible, reimplanting the ureters into the taenia of a sigmoid colon segment in an antirefluxing manner with the sigmoid segment being sutured to the bladder.

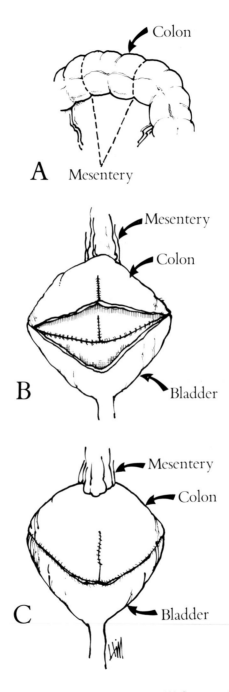

FIGURE 5. Bladder augmentation using colon segment. (A) Segment of colon to be isolated along with its mesentery. (B) After colon segment has been opened along its antimesenteric border, it is sutured to the bladder segment with its mesentery intact. (C) The completed bladder augmentation.

Kass and Koff performed bladder augmentations on 14 patients with neurogenic bladder dysfunction between the ages of 4 and 17 years of age.[18] Thirteen of the 14 children were reported as having stable upper urinary tracts and were continent when adhering to an effective catheterization regimen. One of the 14 children had persistent ureteral reflux after augmentation. Gearhart and coworkers also have reported success with augmentation cystoplasty in the pediatric population.[19]

The majority of patients will initially have difficulty with persistent mucous production from their intestinal segment and will require irrigations along with their intermittent catheterization program in order to remove the mucus. Almost all patients will be required to perform intermittent catheterization after bladder augmentation.

A failure to catheterize frequently in order to prevent distension of the augmented bladder can lead to perforation of the bladder augmentation with subsequent peritonitis and all the ensuing serious complications. Elder and coworkers reported on four cases of perforation of augmented bladders.[20] Periodic electrolyte determinations are required in order to ensure that a hyperchloremic metabolic acidosis does not develop, which is seen when intestinal segments are chronically exposed to urine. Upper urinary tract imaging studies are required periodically to insure adequate drainage of the upper urinary tract. There are also sporadic reported cases of malignancy in augmented bladders arising on the intestinal segment. The long-term risk of developing a malignancy is unknown, but it must be kept in mind during the long-term follow-up period.[21]

The technique of autoaugmentation recently developed by Cartwright and Snow achieves the same goals as bladder augmentation, namely increased bladder capacity with improved bladder wall compliance.[22] The procedure involves stripping away a large segment of the outer muscular wall of the neurogenic bladder from the underlying mucosa. The bladder mucosa is left intact and behaves like a large diverticulum. Early results with this technique are encouraging with the major advantage over bladder augmentation being a much shorter hospitalization time and decreased surgical morbidity.

2. Increasing Outlet Resistance

Despite optimal management with intermittent catheterization, multiple drug therapy, and bladder augmentation, there are patients who will continue to be incontinent because of inadequate bladder outlet resistance. A number of options are available that provide increased outlet resistance, including reconstruction of the bladder neck, insertion of an artificial urinary sphincter, and urethral suspension procedures. All of these options require surgical intervention and all have their own advantages and disadvantages. However, when successful, they all can provide adequate outlet resistance allowing for social continence.

a. Bladder Neck Reconstruction

There are many different types of bladder neck reconstructions, but the most commonly used procedure is the Young-Dees-Leadbetter technique.[23] This technique involves the tubularization of the bladder neck in order to increase outlet resistance. The success of the technique relies on the inherent muscle tone of the bladder neck musculature. Consequently, in those patients with myelodysplasia who have a hypotonic bladder neck and decreased muscular tone secondary to their neurological deficit, tubularization of the bladder neck may not result in adequate outlet resistance. However, Mitchell and Rink reported a greater than 80% success with this technique in patients with neurogenic bladders when combined with bladder augmentation.[24]

A recent innovation in bladder neck reconstruction was introduced by Kropp and Angwafo.[25] Their procedure involves detaching the urethra from the bladder neck and reimplanting the urethra into the bladder neck in a fashion similar to the technique used for implantation of the ureter in patients with vesicoureteral reflux. The use of this procedure requires the use of CIC indefinitely which does not present a problem for most patients with spina bifida.

b. Artificial Urinary Sphincter

The inflatable artificial urinary sphincter was introduced by Scott et al. in 1973.[26] The sphincter has been effectively used in children for a number of years.[27] The sphincter is an artificial device made up of three major components including an inflatable silicone cuff, fluid reservoir, and control pump mechanism. All three components are connected by silicone tubing that allows the fluid in the balloon reservoir to flow through the control pump and into the sphincter cuff. The sphincter cuff is placed around the bladder neck in males and females and may also be placed around the bulbous urethra in older males. The control mechanism is placed in either the scrotum in males or labia majora in females. The balloon reservoir is placed anterior to the peritoneum but under the rectus muscles in the lower abdomen (Figures 6 and 7).

The system works by a hydraulic principle in which the cuff is filled with fluid, thereby occluding the bladder neck until the fluid is pumped out of the cuff by the control pump mechanism into the balloon reservoir allowing evacuation of urine. Although some patients are able to empty their bladder spontaneously, intermittent catheterization is still required in most patients and can be easily performed with an artificial sphincter in place.

Since its inception, the inflatable artificial urinary sphincter has undergone many changes, resulting in a significant improvement in the success rate, where at the present time one can expect at least a 90% success rate in achieving social urinary continence. While certainly an improvement in the management of urinary incontinence in spina bifida, the artificial urinary sphincter is not problem free. Since the artificial sphincter is an artificial device, it is unreasonable to expect that it will function for the entire lifetime of the patient when placed in a child or young adult. Potential problems include

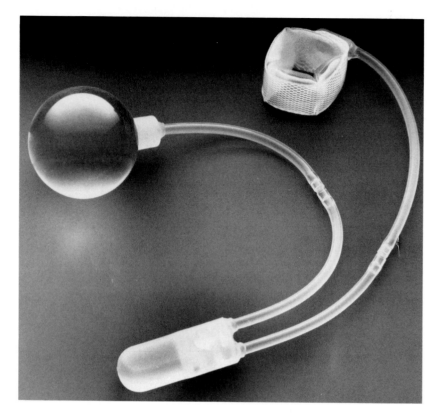

A

FIGURE 6. (A) AMS 800 artificial urinary sphincter and (B) diagram showing device *in situ* in a female with the cuff around the bladder neck. (Courtesy of American Medical Systems, Inc., Minnetonka, MN.)

leakage of the hydraulic fluid through a break anywhere in the device leading to inadequate outlet resistance and subsequent incontinence. Other problems include infection of the device requiring removal of the components. Erosion of the cuff through the bladder neck or of the control pump through the scrotum also requires removal of the components.

Patient selection is important in determining which patients should undergo insertion of an artificial urinary sphincter. The device has been placed in children as young as 5 years of age, but in general, it is preferable to wait until a child has shown enough responsibility and maturity to participate in the management of the sphincter. Enthusiastic patient participation in the care of the sphincter is mandatory. Since the sphincter is extremely successful in preventing urinary incontinence, it is important that the bladder be emptied frequently in order to prevent increased intravesical pressure and subsequent

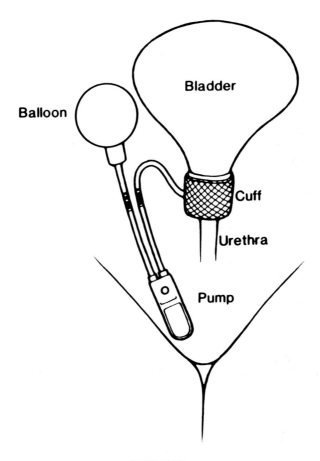

FIGURE 6B.

upper urinary tract deterioration. Preoperative evaluation of the patient is extremely important when considering insertion of an artificial urinary sphincter. Those patients with poor bladder compliance, detrusor hypertonicity, and vesicoureteral reflux will need these underlying problems addressed prior to the insertion of an artificial sphincter.

Depending upon a patient's preoperative evaluation, some patients require bladder augmentation prior to insertion of the sphincter or in combination with sphincter insertion. If bladder compliance is inadequate, an artificial sphincter will hasten the deterioration of the bladder and subsequent upper tract deterioration. Detrussor hypertonicity must be controlled prior to sphincter insertion with either bladder augmentation or anticholinergic medication. Urodynamic studies should be routinely performed preoperatively in order to evaluate bladder wall compliance and the presence of uninhibited contractions. Woodside and McGuire recommend performing urodynamic studies utilizing a balloon catheter to occlude the bladder neck during the urodynamic study in

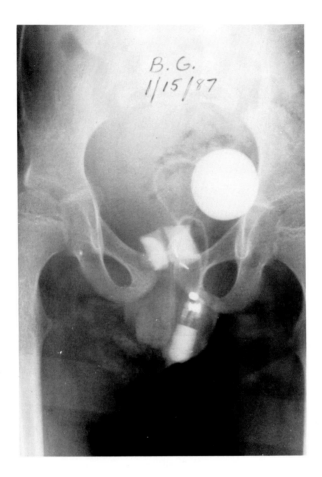

FIGURE 7. Plain X-ray of the artificial urinary sphincter in a teenage male with the cuff around the bladder neck.

order to simulate the effect of an artificial sphincter.[28] Using this technique, bladder wall compliance in the presence of an artificial sphincter can be simulated. Gonzalez and Sheldon reported on their experience with artificial urinary sphincters in children and showed good success on patients who were evaluated over the long term.[29]

c. Vesical Neck Suspension

Vesical neck suspension procedures have become more popular as an alternative to bladder neck reconstruction and the artificial urinary sphincter. The most popular techniques include the suprapubic endoscopic vesical neck suspension or the use of a pubovaginal sling. Woodside and Borden reported success in treating urinary incontinence in myelodysplastic girls by using the endoscopic technique.[30] The pubovaginal sling as described by McGuire and co-workers involves the use of a strip of rectus fascia which is placed on either side of the urethra and tied over the anterior fascia.[31] Eight girls with myelodysplasia were dry on intermittent catheterization after the pubovaginal sling. They reported an increase of 12 to 15 cm of water over the preoperative bladder leak point pressure. Success with this procedure is limited to females at this time because of the difficulty in adequately suspending the male prostatic urethra with these techniques. When successful, the sling and endoscopic suspension procedures are preferable to an insertion of an artificial urinary sphincter since no artificial device is required.

3. Urinary Diversion

In the past, many patients with spina bifida underwent urinary diversion, mainly with the ileal conduit because of recurrent urinary tract infection or persistent urinary incontinence. The introduction of CIC radically changed the treatment of children with spina bifida and eliminated the routine use of permanent urinary diversions.

a. Temporary Urinary Diversion

Temporary urinary diversion with a cutaneous vesicostomy is still utilized in newborns or small infants who require CIC but in whom frequent catheterization is not possible or in those patients with urinary tract deterioration unresponsive to catheterization because of a small capacity, noncompliant bladder. The vesicostomy is used as a temporizing procedure until the patient is older and can more easily undergo bladder augmentation. The Blocksom technique for cutaneous vesicostomy utilizes a small transverse incision halfway between the pubis and umbilicus and requires exposure of the bladder dome near the urachal remnant for the location of the stoma.[32] This technique reduces the incidence of vesical prolapse. Cohen et al. reported an incidence of vesical prolapse in 25% of their patients, and 42% had problems with dermatitis.[33] The vesicostomy is closed at a time when CIC may be more acceptable usually around age 3 to 4.

b. Permanent Urinary Diversion

Permanent urinary diversion is avoided as much as possible and has become an acceptable treatment only when all other options are exhausted. The standard form of urinary diversion in patients with spina bifida was the ileal conduit, which involved isolating a segment of ileum and anastomosing the ureters into the proximal end of the ileum. This type of urinary diversion allows free reflux of urine into the upper urinary tract. The disadvantages of this type of urinary tract management included the need for continual application of an ostomy bag, and all of the associated social problems that accompany ostomy appliances. Long-term results of the ileal conduit urinary diversion in children reveals this type of urinary tract management to be less than optimal from a medical standpoint. Shapiro and co-workers studied 90 children who underwent ileal conduit urinary diversion for nonmalignant disease.[34] Over half of these patients had spina bifida. They found that stomal obstruction was the most common complication occurring in 38% of patients. Ureteroileal obstruction occurred in 22%. Two thirds of their patients required some form of ileal loop revision in a 10 to 16 year follow-up. Of the 144 renal units studied, 26 deteriorated during the period of time that was analyzed by the study.

Because of the refluxing nature of the ileal loop urinary diversion, the use of a colon conduit with nonrefluxing ureteral anatomoses has been recommended as an alternative. Altwein et al. followed 64 children who underwent colon conduit urinary diversion because of complications of spina bifida and found that 9.4% had early postoperative surgical complications while 14.5% had late surgical complications.[35] Of the renal units studied, 91% appeared normal during their follow-up period. Although the nonrefluxing colon conduit is superior to the refluxing ileal conduit, there is still a significant deterioration rate and the problem of the ostomy appliance is still present.

c. Continent Urinary Diversion

In an attempt to provide a suitable alternative to the ileal conduit for those patients who require permanent urinary diversion, different forms of continent urinary diversions have been developed. The advantage of the continent urinary diversion is the elimination of an ostomy appliance. Regardless of the type of continent diversion used, the patient is required to catheterize a urinary reservoir through a continent stoma located on the abdominal wall.

The Koch ileal reservoir utilizes a length of ileum which is reconfigured to create a large pouch acting as the reservoir which is attached to 2 limbs of ileum which are intususcepted.[36] One limb is used for the catheterizable continent stoma, while the other limb is used for the ureteral-ileal anatomoses. Because of the intususception, this is a nonrefluxing type of reservoir.

Although this technique has been utilized mainly in adults with bladder cancer, it does have applications in patients with spina bifida who require urinary diversion. There are a number of other types of continent diversions, some of which use the ileal cecal segment. The main qualifications that a continent urinary diversion must fulfill are that it must be a low pressure reservoir, and that it must have nonrefluxing ureteral anatomoses. Since these procedures are relatively new, the long-term results are pending and this should be of concern to surgeons implementing these diversions in young patients who have a long life expectancy. The immediate surgical complication risks are much higher with these procedures than in comparison to the ileal loop diversion. The long-term complication rates are still unknown.

There is a subgroup of patients who cannot be catheterized through the urethra for a variety of reasons, including a tortuous urethra secondary to catheter induced false passages. Since it is preferable to keep the urinary tract intact and eliminate the need for a urinary diversion, the ability to catheterize the bladder through a continent stoma rather than the urethra would be beneficial. Mitrofanoff described a technique involving the use of the appendix as a continent stoma that is attached to the bladder in a nonrefluxing manner.[37] This allows for the catheterization of the bladder through the continent stoma. This idea has been taken one step further, whereby the distal ureter is brought out to the skin as a continent stoma. The proximal ureter can be connected to the contralateral ureter through a transureterostomy.

4. Urinary Undiversion

Since the standard treatment for many patients with spina bifida in the past was permanent urinary diversion with an ileal conduit, there is subsequently a large group of patients who are candidates for urinary undiversion given the recent developments in the surgical treatment of the neurogenic bladder. With the development of bladder augmentation, the artificial urinary sphincter, bladder neck reconstructive techniques, and intermittent catheterization, most patients who have previously undergone urinary diversion can be successfully undiverted. Patient selection is extremely important, since many patients who have been successfully diverted for a number of years are reluctant to give up their type of urinary drainage and should not be coerced into undergoing urinary undiversion unless they have a high level of enthusiasm for the procedure. Prior to urinary undiversion, a patient must undergo radiographic and urodynamic evaluation in order to properly assess the underlying anatomy and degree of outlet resistance. It is very important that a patient be able to perform CIC prior to a diversion and they must show motivation and compliance with the recommended regimen. The patient should be aware that there is the possibility of urinary incontinence, and in some cases, the patients have desired a return to permanent urinary diversion after undiversion. Bauer et al. reported a successful outcome in the majority of their patients with spina bifida who underwent urinary undiversion.[38]

E. Electrical Stimulation of the Bladder

Electrical stimulation of the bladder by either an anal plug or implanted electrode has been shown to be of limited use in patients with spina bifida. Godec and Cass provided electrical stimulation of the bladder through an anal plug.[39] They had very limited long-term success in treating incontinence. Wheatley et al. implanted electrode wires on the lateral aspect of the bladder in the region of the neurovascular pedicles.[40] The electrode wires were connected to a bladder stimulator placed in a subcutaneous pocket in the lower abdomen. Satisfactory results were obtained in 3 of 8 children, but the long-term functioning of the units was poor. With the success of intermittent catheterization and the more successful surgical alternatives available at this time, electronic stimulation of the pelvic floor musculature is presently not a frequently used modality.

F. Circumcision and Spina Bifida

Although there is some debate on this issue, routine circumcision in male patients with spina bifida should be discouraged. The prepuce protects the neurologically insensitive glans penis from irritation and the dermatitis frequently seen with persistent incontinence. Some children, however, do require circumcision because of the development of a persistently inflamed prepuce that can lead to phimosis and the inability to perform intermittent catheterization.

VII. SEXUALITY AND SPINA BIFIDA

The majority of patients with spina bifida can have an active sex life, and in the majority of patients, pregnancy is a realistic possibility. Cass et al. reported on the sexual function and childbearing experience of 47 patients with spina bifida who were 16 or more years old.[41] Their studies showed that 11 of 12 men studied were able to have full erections with 9 having ejaculation and orgasm. Of 35 women surveyed, 17 experienced sexual intercourse, whereas 12 of 35 women became pregnant. Because of the increased risk of developing a neural tube malformation, genetic counseling is advised. It is important that the message be conveyed to young adults with spina bifida that they can, in most cases, have a satisfactory sex life.

REFERENCES

1. **Kroovand, R. L.,** Myelomeningocele, in *Campbell's Urology,* Vol. 2, 5th ed., Walsh, P. C., Gittes, R. F., Perlmutter, A. D., and Stamey, T. A., Eds., W. B. Saunders, Philadelphia, 1986, 2205.
2. **Roberts, J. B. M.,** Congenital anomalies of the urinary tract and their association with spina bifida, *Br. J. Urol.,* 33, 309, 1961.
3. **Fernbach, S. K. and Davis, T. M.,** The abnormal renal axis in children with spina bifida and gibbus deformity — the pseudohorseshoe kidney, *J. Urol.,* 136, 1258, 1986.
4. **Kass, E. J., Koff, S. A., Diokno, A. C., and Lapides, J., Jr.,** The significance of bacilluria in children on long term intermittent catheterization, *J. Urol.,* 126, 223, 1981.
5. **McGuire, E. J., Woodside, J. R., Borden, T. A., and Weiss, R. M.,** Prognostic value of urodynamic testing in myelodysplastic patients, *J. Urol.,* 126, 205, 1981.
6. **Chiaramonte, R. M., Horowitz, E. M., Kaplan, G. W., and Brock, W. A.,** Implications of hydronephrosis in the newborn with myelodysplasia, *J. Urol.,* 136, 427, 1986.
7. **Bauer, S. B.,** Early evaluation and management of children with spina bifida, in *Urologic Surgery in Neonates and Young Infants,* King, L. R., Ed., W. B. Saunders, Philadelphia, 1988, 261.
8. **Enrile, G. B. and Crooks, J. K.,** Clean intermittent catheterization for home management in children with myelomeningocele, *Clin. Pediatr.,* 19, 743, 1980.
9. **Bauer, S. B., Hallett, N., Koshbin, S., Lebowitz, R. L., Winston, K. R., Gibson, S., Colodny, A. H., and Retik, A. B.,** Predictive value of urodynamic evaluation of newborns with myelodysplasia, *JAMA,* 252, 650, 1984.
10. **Gaum, L. D., Wese, F. X., Alton, D. J., Hardy, B. E., and Churchill, B. M.,** Radiologic investigation of the urinary tract in the neonate with myelomeningocele, *J. Urol.,* 127, 510, 1982.

11. **Whitaker, R. H.,** Methods of assessing obstruction in dilated ureter, *Br. J. Urol.,* 45, 15, 1973.

12. **Sidi, A. A., Dykstra, D. D., and Gonzalez, R.,** The value of urodynamic testing the management of neonates with myelodysplasia, a prospective study, *J. Urol.,* 135, 90, 1986.

13. **Spindel, M. R., Bauer, S. B., Dyro, F. M., Krarup, C., Khoshbin, S., Winston, K. R., Lebowitz, R. L., Colodny, A. H., and Retik, A. B.,** The changing neurourologic lesion in myelodysplasia, *JAMA,* 258, 1630, 1987.

14. **Lapides, J., Diokno, A. C., Silber, S. J., and Lowe, B.,** Clean intermittent self-catheterization in the treatment of urinary tract disease, *J. Urol.,* 107, 458, 1972.

15. **Kass, E. J., McHugh, T., and Diokno, A. C.,** Intermittent catheterization in children less than six years old, *J. Urol.,* 121, 792, 1979.

16. **Ehrlich, O. and Brem, A. S.,** A prospective comparison of urinary tract infections in patients treated with either clean intermittent catheterization or urinary diversion, *Pediatrics,* 70, 665, 1982.

17. **Hilwa, N. and Perlmutter, A. D.,** The role of adjunctive drug therapy for intermittent catheterization and self-catheterization in children with vesical dysfunction, *J. Urol.,* 119, 551, 1978.

18. **Kass, E. J. and Koff, S. A.,** Bladder augmentation in the pediatric neuropathic bladder, *J. Urol.,* 129, 552, 1983.

19. **Gearhart, J. P., Albertsen, P. C., Marshall, F. F., and Jeff, R. D.,** Pediatric applications of augmentation cystoplasty: the Johns Hopkins experience, *J. Urol.,* 136, 430, 1986.

20. **Elder, J. S., Snyder, H. M., Hulbert, W. C., and Duckett, J. W.,** Perforation of augmented bladder in patients undergoing clean intermittent catheterization, *J. Urol.,* 140, 1159, 1988.

21. **Filmer, R. B.,** Malignant tumors arising in bladder augmentations, and ileal and colon conduits, *Soc. Pediatr. Urol. Newsl.,* October 24, 1986.

22. **Cartwright, P. C. and Snow, B. W.,** Autoaugmentation: early clinical experience, presented at the American Academy of Pediatrics Annual Meeting, October 15 to 17, 1988.

23. **Leadbetter, G. W., Jr.,** Surgical correction of total urinary incontinence, *J. Urol.,* 91, 261, 1964.

24. **Mitchell, M. D. and Rink, R. C.,** Urinary diversion and undiversion, *Urol. Clin. North Am.,* 12, 111, 1985.

25. **Kropp, K. A. and Angwafo, F. F.,** Urethral lengthening and reimplantation for neurogenic incontinence in children, *J. Urol.,* 135, 533, 1986.

26. **Scott, F. B., Bradley, W. E., and Timm, G. W.,** Treatment of urinary incontinence by implantable prosthetic sphincter, *Urology,* 1, 252, 1973.

27. **Barrett, D. M. and Furlow, W. L.,** Artificial urinary sphincter in children, in *Clinical Pediatric Urology,* Vol. 1, 2nd ed., Kelalis, P. P., King, L. R., and Belman, A. B., Eds., W. B. Saunders, Philadelphia, 1985, 345.

28. **Woodside, J. R. and McGuire, E. J.,** Technique for detection of detrusor hypertonia in the presence of urethral sphincteric incompetence, *J. Urol.,* 127, 740, 1982.

29. **Gonzalez, R. and Sheldon, C. A.,** Artificial sphincters in children with neurogenic bladders: long term results, *J. Urol.,* 128, 1270, 1982.

30. **Woodside, J. R. and Borden, T. A.,** Suprapubic endoscopic vesical neck suspension for the management of urinary incontinence in myelodysplastic girls, *J. Urol.,* 135, 97, 1986.

31. **McGuire, E. J., Wang, C., Usitalo, H., and Sarastano, J.,** Modified pubovaginal sling in girls with myelodysplasia, *J. Urol.,* 135, 94, 1986.

32. **Duckett, J. W.,** Cutaneous vesicostomy in childhood, the Blocksom technique, *Urol. Clin. North Am.,* 1, 485, 1974.

33. **Cohen, J. S., Harbach, L. B., and Kaplan, G. W.,** Cutaneous vesicostomy for temporary urinary diversion in infants with neurogenic bladder dysfunction, *J. Urol.,* 119, 120, 1978.

34. **Shapiro, S. R., Lebowitz, R., and Colodny, A. H.,** Fate of 90 children with ileal conduit urinary diversion a decade later: analysis of complications, pyelography, renal function and bacteriology, *J. Urol.,* 114, 289, 1975.

35. **Altwein, J. E., Jones, U., and Hohenfellner, R.,** Longterm follow-up of children with colon conduit urinary diversion and ureterosigmoid, *J. Urol.,* 118, 832, 1977.

36. **Boyd, S. D., Skinner, D. G., and Lieskovsky, G.,** The Kock Continent Ileal Urinary Reservoir, AUA Update Series, Vol. 4, Lesson 38, American Urological Association, 1985.

37. **Duckett, J. W. and Snyder, H. M.,** Use of the Mitrofanoff principle in urinary reconstruction, *Urol. Clin. North Am.,* 13, 271, 1986.

38. **Bauer, S. B., Colodny, A. H., Hallet, M., Khoshbin, S., and Retik, A. B.,** Urinary undiversion in myelodysplasia and criteria for selection and predictive value of urodynamic evaluation, *J. Urol.,* 124, 89, 1980.

39. **Godec, C. J. and Cass, A. S.,** Electrical stimulation for incontinence in myelomeningocele, *J. Urol.,* 120, 729, 1978.

40. **Wheatley, J. K., Woodard, J. R., and Parrott, T. S.,** Electronic bladder stimulation in the management of children with myelomeningocele, *J. Urol.,* 127, 283, 1982.

41. **Cass, A. S., Bloom, B. A., and Luxenberg, M.,** Sexual function in adults with myelomeningocele, *J. Urol.,* 136, 425, 1986.

Chapter 9

REACHING ADULTHOOD — THE LONG-TERM PSYCHOSOCIAL ADJUSTMENT OF CHILDREN WITH SPINA BIFIDA

Lynda Dallyn and Carolynne Garrison-Jones

TABLE OF CONTENTS

Due to medical advancements, many children with spina bifida are now living longer, and subsequently, their psychosocial needs have become greater. Multiple issues need to be addressed and interventions developed in order to assist these children in their struggle for independence and transition into adulthood. In this chapter we examine the challenges presently facing the young adult with spina bifida and present a conceptual model that summarizes factors that may be influential in facilitating more positive long-term psychosocial outcomes for the child with spina bifida. This framework emphasizes that successful transition into adulthood is intimately related to a complex interplay between the multiple systems within which the child with spina bifida has been enmeshed during his or her lifetime. The final goal of this chapter is to offer guidelines for families, health care providers, other professionals, and public policy makers that might be useful in helping the child with spina bifida achieve a more autonomous, productive, and rewarding life as an adult.

I. CHALLENGES FACING THE YOUNG ADULT WITH SPINA BIFIDA

It is well established that throughout the life span, children with chronic illnesses such as spina bifida are at greater risk for problems in areas of psychological and social functioning.[3,31] From the first breath of life, the child with spina bifida faces some of the most complex and difficult challenges that accompany any congenital defect. Beginning at birth with the initial struggle to stay alive until the transition into adulthood, the affected child must cope with a variety of obstacles that have the potential for interfering with successful psychosocial adaptation. Each developmental phase presents its own set of accompanying stresses that both children and their families must overcome. For example, the newborn and infant are often hospitalized and separated from parents. This absence of the child from the home potentially affects the parent/child bonding process and the child's development of basic trust. Frequently, the curious preschooler is held back from exploring and learning about the world around him or her because of limited mobility related to orthopedic problems. Also, as these children enter school, they often experience peer ridicule and rejection due to the visibility of their handicap.

By far, the most challenging periods for the person with spina bifida are adolescence and young adulthood. Many authors point to adolescence as a time for increased risk of psychological distress.[36] Adolescence has been characterized as a time when significant biological, cognitive, emotional, and social changes take place.[8] Separation from parents, a search for self-identity, increased responsibility and independence, planning for a future career, and the establishment of meaningful interpersonal relationships are among the goals of this time.[13,36] For most adolescents, the experience is one marked by intense insecurity, anxiety, depression, and self-doubt. Because of the additional coping requirements, the handicapped child will perceive this period as being even more stressful.

A review of the literature pertaining to the emotional adjustment of children with spina bifida and chronic illness more generally finds a linear increase in the occurrence of psychosocial problems with age.[11,31] In a study of 3 year olds, no significant differences emerged when children with spina bifida were compared with a nonhandicapped control group on such variables as behavioral problems and anxiety.[3] During primary school years, children with spina bifida have been reported to show some increased feelings of anxiety and fearfulness, although not strikingly different than normal populations.[3] However, by early adolescence, children with physical handicaps, spina bifida included, show very high rates of symptomatology suggestive of psychological disturbance.[3,9-11,42] Several of these authors comment that the increased problems noted during this period reflect both the cumulative effects of stresses incurred during childhood in combination with the increased coping demands of adolescence. Also significant is the observation that in the few studies of children with spina bifida, there is a consistent finding that these children more frequently display symptomatology of an "internalizing" nature rather than antisocial or acting out behavior.[3,6,9,40] Although the reliability and significance of this finding needs to be borne out in future research, these studies suggest that young adolescents with spina bifida experience a substantial amount of anxiety that may be kept private. A recent study addressing the continuity of behavioral and emotional disturbance in physically handicapped children aged 6 to 18 found that unlike their nonhandicapped counterparts, children with spina bifida were among those physically handicapped children who showed persistent emotional and social problems over a 5-year period.[6]

The outlook becomes more bleak when current data pertaining to the psychosocial and vocational adjustment of the young adult with spina bifida are considered. The few studies that specifically focus on or include young adults with spina bifida point to an increased occurrence of such problems as depression, anxiety, low self-esteem, social isolation, and unemployment.[1-3,7,41] In 1982, Anderson and Clark,[2] found in their study of young people with both spina bifida and cerebral palsy that many of these individuals had disturbed family relationships, significant fears about the future, felt a general lack of control over their lives, and had very little knowledge of community support services. The most significant indicator of psychological distress, however, was the pervasive social isolation experienced by these youth and a perceived lack of supportive interpersonal relationships. The level of social activity in this study was found to be related to the degree of handicap.

With regard to vocational adjustment, several studies have found very high rates of unemployment among young adults with spina bifida.[3,7,39] Estimates range from 30 to 60%, and increase with the severity of mental handicap. For those individuals who do receive employment, there are frequently long delays to job placement and considerable anxiety about their usefulness and security. Also, few young adults with spina bifida are likely to enroll in higher education programs. Tew,[39] in a longitudinal study of spina bifida patients born between 1964 and 1966 in South Wales, found them to score significantly poorer on national examinations than control subjects and indicated that 94% were unlikely to enter college. Most disturbing, however, is the finding that many of these young adults continue to live at home, dependent on their parents.[2,3,7]

The emotional, social, and biological needs of the young adult with spina bifida are essentially the same as those for nonhandicapped persons. As with any emerging adult, the person with spina bifida strives to satisfy a basic need for love, acceptance, and a sense of self-worth. Equally important is the need for meaningful family, social, and intimate relationships. Finally, most young adults yearn for independence, financial security, and an opportunity to express talents and abilities. Perhaps the greatest challenge facing young adults with spina bifida is society's unpreparedness to meet the many emotional, social, academic, and vocational needs that they present. Society's attitude toward and willingness to assist the disabled person has not changed significantly over time as might be expected of a progressive mankind. Handicapped individuals continue to be misunderstood and discriminated against and their needs often go unaddressed. Presently, employment opportunities and social outlets are not readily available and professionals often discontinue their involvement when the child completes high school. It seems unrealistic to expect that these youths should live independently of those support systems that were available during pediatric years. These obstacles must be overcome if young adults with spina bifida are to achieve a quality of life they deserve.

Given that persons with spina bifida are now living well into adulthood combined with our understanding of the negative psychosocial consequences that accompany this disorder, it becomes very important for us to begin identifying factors that play a role in altering the risk of long-term adjustment problems for this population. Although there has been much focus given to those with spina bifida who do experience adjustment problems, there are many others who display very successful adaptation. An important question then arises concerning the existence of variables that might operate in a protective fashion to moderate the probability of negative psychosocial outcomes. This chapter presents a conceptual framework that addresses this issue.

II. CONCEPTUAL MODEL OF PSYCHOSOCIAL ADJUSTMENT

For the child with spina bifida, successful psychosocial adaptation in adulthood is dependent on the complex interplay between a number of different factors. Medical variables, individual characteristics and competencies of the child, family and social relationships, environmental support systems, and broader societal values and beliefs directly and indirectly impact on long-term adjustment outcomes. It is proposed that in addition to their direct impact on autonomy and overall psychosocial functioning, these domains reciprocally influence one another. For example, individual child characteristics influence family and peer relationship factors. The quality of these interactions, in turn, play a role in determining individual child characteristics. Similarly, education and community resources impact on both individual and family characteristics. Both individuals and families, however, are also able to influence educational and community systems. There are myriad ways that each domain might mutually influence each other and impact on the long-term psychosocial adjustment of the spina bifida patient (Figure 1). Many authors have highlighted the importance of adopting an ecological perspective when considering issues relating to the adjustment of children with spina bifida and chronic illness more generally.[3,5,11] As is true with all persons, the child with spina bifida will display greater or lesser difficulty transitioning to adulthood depending on his or her individual capabilities, competencies, and experiences in the social environment.

There have been virtually no empirical research studies that have investigated characteristics of the individual and social environment that are predictive of successful and unsuccessful adaptation of spina bifida patients. Much of the literature pertaining to this issue is theoretical in nature and employs correlational, cross-sectional designs. While prospective, longitudinal methods are superior in their ability to detect direct, causal relationships, the existing literature does provide a starting point from which to begin identifying potentially important variables. Below we examine selected variables that may hold particular importance for the development of autonomy and healthy long-term psychosocial functioning of the child with spina bifida. Medical factors, individual child characteristics, social relationship factors, and social-environmental variables are discussed and their interrelationship with one another is highlighted.

A. Medical Considerations

For all children born with spina bifida, there exist associated malformations and medical problems that vary in severity depending on the level of the spinal lesion.[29] Perhaps the most serious of these problems are hydrocephalus, lower body paralysis, and bowel and bladder incontinence.[29] The combination of these conditions has a major impact on the child's overall well-being in two interrelated ways. First, the physical involvement of spina bifida restricts many of the child's bodily functions, frequently causes pain, and requires regular medical care and surgical intervention in order to achieve some semblance of a normal life. Hence, the affected person potentially spends a large portion of his or her early life in clinics and hospitals, away from the family. Second, these related physical problems have a direct influence on the child's long-term psychosocial adjustment. For example, hydrocephalus typically affects the child's cognitive ability; lower body paralysis may prohibit mobility and social

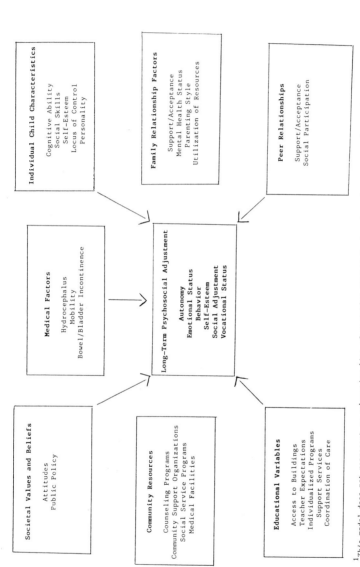

FIGURE 1.   Ecological model of psychosocial adjustment in spina bifida patients.[1]

[1]This model does not represent an exhaustive list of variables thought to impact on long-term psychosocial adjustment.

interaction; and bowel and bladder incontinence may cause embarrassment and low self-esteem.

B. Individual Child Characteristics

Individual characteristics and competencies of the person refer to the resources inherent within the human being and encompass such variables as cognitive functioning, personality and temperament, personal coping skills, self-esteem, and locus of control. It is proposed that these factors in combination with a variety of other influences, including the child's family and social relationships, operate to determine the risk for psychosocial problems during the course of development and in adulthood. It is important to recognize that in addition to their direct impact on psychosocial functioning, these domains also exert a reciprocal influence on each other. For example, if the child with spina bifida possesses numerous positive qualities such as above-average cognitive ability and social skills, in all likelihood, this will have a positive influence on his or her family system, social relationships, and prospects for overall achievement. The child's individual strengths can operate to promote positive social relationships which offer support and a decreased probability of social isolation.

1. Cognitive Ability

A number of studies suggest that children with spina bifida, on the average, display lowered cognitive ability when compared with their nonhandicapped counterparts.[3,39] Although the IQ distribution is skewed toward the lower end for spina bifida patients, there is some variability in performance, particularly between those individuals with and without hydrocephalus.[3,39] It has also been noted that while individuals with spina bifida typically display problems in areas of perceptual-motor ability, numerical reasoning, and attention, they show some variation in the pattern of cognitive deficits. Tew and Laurence[41] in their longitudinal study of spina bifida patients, found a very strong relationship between IQ at age 5 and 16 and concluded that it is frequently possible to predict eventual academic success at school entry.

While there are no empirical studies addressing the relationship between cognitive status and psychosocial functioning in spina bifida patients, it is suspected that cognitive ability plays a significant role in long-term adjustment. A child's cognitive ability is directly related to performance in the educational arena which, in turn, has implications for vocational adjustment and independence in adulthood. It is also likely that this variable impacts on a variety of other factors including self-help skills, self-esteem, problem solving ability, development and maintenance of social relationships, and parental and sibling adjustment.

2. Social Skills

Although there has been much discussion about the social skills of individuals with spina bifida, very little is actually known about their interpersonal ability. Many authors have commented that persons with spina bifida display an increased tendency toward passivity, immaturity, and dependence in their social interactions. However, virtually no empirical research has investigated differences between spina bifida populations and nonhandicapped controls on these or other relevant variables. Given the orthopedic problems often experienced by many individuals with spina bifida, it seems reasonable to expect that there would be some adaptive component of dependence in their interpersonal relationships. However, there is no evidence to indicate whether this attribute is representative of a broader interactional style. Similarly, considering the cognitive deficits that often accompany this medical condition, it appears likely that there would be a higher incidence of social immaturity. Because a percentage of children with hydrocephalus often demonstrate excessive verbalization, often referred to as the "cocktail party syndrome", their verbal interactions may be confusing to others and may present the false hope of more meaningful social interaction.[20] This may lead to recurring social rejection.

Given that interpersonal skills are the gateway through which social relationships are established and maintained, they take on particular significance as mediators of support resources in the individual's life. Social skills also greatly influence a variety of other factors including family attitude, the degree of one's negotiation for environmental support resources, and self-esteem. Therefore, to the degree that the child with spina bifida possesses strengths in the area of social skill, his or her prospects for more positive long-term adjustment will increase.

3. Self-Esteem

Self-esteem is an extremely valuable personal resource that no doubt plays a key role in insulating the individual with chronic illness from the numerous stresses and challenges that are presented during the course of development. A number of authors have suggested that individuals with spina bifida are more inclined to exhibit low self-esteem.[30] However, the few empirical studies that have been conducted have found either conflicting results or no significant differences between this group and relevant comparison groups.[24,30] Pearson and co-workers[30] did find a negative correlation between the length of time the child spent in the hospital during the first 6 years of life and self-esteem at age 12. These authors indicate that this relationship may, in part, be attributable to early disruption in the parent/child relationship.

Recent literature highlights the importance of viewing self-esteem as a multidimensional concept.[35] In addition to global self-esteem, which can be defined as the general feeling of self-worth, also important are feelings of self-esteem relating to specific domains such as social and academic skill and body image. Perhaps measures of global self-esteem are not reflective of particular problem areas for those with spina bifida. It is possible that significant differences between this population and nonhandicapped controls only emerge when comparisons are made on more specific dimensions of self-esteem. Considering the orthopedic problems and physical limitations that often accompany spina bifida, it would appear that further investigation in the area of body image would be particularly important. Also, information regarding the role an individual's appraisal of his or her handicap plays in psychosocial adjustment would be a valuable area for further investigation. It is encouraging, however, that preliminary findings seem to indicate that spina bifida patients are not globally compromised in the area of self-esteem.

4. Locus of Control

Locus of control is an expression used to describe a dimension of personality functioning that reflects the degree to which one perceives himself as having control over the environment and significant life events.[23] Internal locus of control refers to a belief in the ability to impact the environment and control important events while external locus of control reflects a perceived inability to prevail over one's environment and manage significant stressors. It has generally been found that those with an internal locus of control take a more active approach when attempting to manage stress and resolve problems, while individuals with an external locus of control are more apt to perceive stress and react more negatively to problem situations.[23] A large number of studies identify a strong correlation between external locus of control and psychological distress, particularly depression.[4]

Given the challenges facing children with spina bifida throughout life, it seems reasonable to presume that their experience in the world will, to some degree, encourage an external locus of control orientation. However, there have been no studies to date that assess possible group differences between spina bifida and nonhandicapped control populations. It seems reasonable to surmise that to the extent that the person with spina bifida adopts an internal locus of control orientation, he or she will be less at risk for developing psychosocial problems in adulthood.

As a summary, in the previous section, several variables pertaining to the individual were proposed to play an important role in the psychosocial adjustment of those with spina bifida throughout the life span. These variables are among a host of factors presumed to have particular significance in long-term adjustment outcomes. Other individual characteristics such as coping style, problem solving ability, and self-help behaviors are also potentially influential factors in adjustment. It is important to recognize that not only will these attributes mutually interact with one another, but they will also directly and indirectly impact on other systems impinging on the individual.

C. Familial and Social Relationship Factors

Many authors addressing adjustment concerns related to pediatric chronic illness have described the reciprocal effect families and children have on one another.[17,25] Families are affected in a number of ways by chronic illness of one of its members, and in turn, play a significant role in influencing the overall adaptation processes of that family member. Parents typically experience significant distress and a range of conflicting feelings upon the birth of a child with spina bifida.[29] Several authors have discussed the fact that parents of chronically ill children must cope with stressful daily circumstances including caretaking responsibilities, demanding treatment schedules, increased expenses, and career restrictions.[28,44] Under these circumstances, parents often experience great difficulty accepting the disabled child.

Several recent studies have found that for the most part many families with children who have spina bifida are able to cope adequately and adapt in ways that are functional.[18] A recent study of nonretarded spina bifida patients, which also included a sample of nondisabled children and their parents, found that those families with children who have spina bifida "do not differ from matched controls in parenting attitude, marital adjustment, perception of child behavior, child self-concept, stress, and overall family functioning."[37] Kazak[16] concludes that the differences between families with and without a disabled child may be fewer than previously suggested.

The family is probably the most significant source of emotional support for an individual.[34] Anderson and Spain,[3] based on a review of literature pertaining to young adults with spina bifida, found that parental reaction to a child's disability and method used for coping is the most critical factor in the child's adjustment. Each family has certain characteristics and informal rules that significantly impact on the child's way of thinking and behaving. The cumulative positive and negative experiences within the family context have an overall effect on the psychosocial adjustment of the young adult with spina bifida. In the discussion that follows, we examine familial variables that are most likely to affect long-term psychological and social functioning. It is important to note that much of the previous research in this field is unreliable and often complicated by methodological flaws.[16]

1. Family Support and Acceptance

Parental attitudes about and perceptions of the child will have a powerful impact on the child's adjustment throughout the life span.[22,29] Families who are unaccepting and unsupportive may interfere with the development of positive self-esteem and coping skills. In contrast, families who are accepting, who emphasize the child's talents and abilities and who assist the child in developing coping skills, are much more effective in helping the child attain positive self-esteem as well as increased independence in adulthood.[29] Numerous authors have highlighted the importance of open communication among family members, and there is some suggestion that the presence of a confiding relationship between a parent and the youth with spina bifida may help prevent the occurrence of emotional adjustment problems.[3,11]

2. Mental Health Status of Family Members

The presence of an individual with chronic illness often creates a significant amount of stress within families which may then contribute to problems of emotional functioning among family members.[11] To the degree that parents and siblings experience mental health problems, the person with spina bifida is at increased risk for developing adjustment problems.[33]

Numerous studies report high rates of emotional distress and depressive symptomatology among mothers of youth with spina bifida.[3,15-18,42,43] These articles elaborate that stress experienced by mothers is typically related to severity of the handicap, caretaking responsibilities such as management of bowel/bladder incontinence, and issues related to mobility. One study found that increased maternal depression among mothers may be related to having an older disabled child than one who is younger.[16]

Given the documented evidence of high levels of parenting stress in families of children with spina bifida, it might be automatically assumed that the stability of the marital relationship in these families is usually compromised. However, several studies have found that marital satisfaction among parents of children with spina bifida does not significantly differ from that of couples with nonhandicapped children.[18] Kolin et al.[21] "found that the length of marriage before the birth of the handicapped child was an important factor in predicting the marital outcome: couples who had been married for at least five years experienced fewer difficulties that those who had been married for a shorter time."[17] Interestingly, Kazak and Marvin[18] found that higher levels of marital satisfaction exist in families whose children with spina bifida are more severely handicapped.[16,17]

The adaptation among siblings of children with spina bifida is best summarized by Tew and Laurence[43] who found this group to be four times more likely to have significant adjustment problems than siblings of a control group.[11,12]

3. Parenting Style

Many parents of children with spina bifida or chronic illnesses are often described as being overprotective and indulgent.[38] This behavior is apt to interfere with the developmental skill necessary for independent functioning. Often parents unconsciously adopt a child rearing style that meets their emotional needs rather than those of their child. In a study of youth with spina bifida, Anderson and Spain[3] observed an overly close bond between mothers and the affected child.

Presently, very little research has addressed the issue of whether there might be certain parenting approaches that reduce the risk of long-term psychosocial adjustment problems among youths with spina bifida. It may be that variables such as parental involvement, appropriate limit setting, consistent discipline, guidance regarding future career, encouragement of independence, and realistic expectations of academic performance and behavior are particularly important in parenting a child with a physical handicap.

4. Utilization of Informal Support Resources

Given the many needs presented by children with spina bifida there is little doubt that affected families require social support in order to effectively cope. However, recent literature suggests that these families often experience a great amount of social isolation.[14] Kazak and Marvin[18] found that the parents of children with spina bifida had fewer supports than parents of nonhandicapped children. Also, their social support networks usually contained more family members than friendships and they were prone to rely heavily on these family members for a variety of support functions. Despite the fact that these parents were observed to have small social networks, the quality of perceived support did not differ from that of normal control group subjects.

It is certainly intuitively logical that to the degree that families are able to access and utilize support offered by extended family members and friends, they will be less vulnerable to the effects of stress that often accompany the presence of a child with spina bifida in the home. Parents who feel support from relatives and friends may be more able to relate in a positive fashion to their child and offer structure needed for normal development.

5. Peer Relationships

The child's experience in the social arena during the course of development will also play a role in short- and long-term psychosocial adjustment. While it is recognized that individual characteristics of the child such as interpersonal skill and cognitive ability will determine the nature of peer relationships, interpersonal interactions with peers will, in turn, influence the child's social skills, self-esteem, and feelings of belonging. Satisfying peer relationships and the need for social participation becomes particularly important during adolescence and adulthood. The absence of close interpersonal relationships and social involvement on the part of the child with spina bifida is likely to result in an increased risk of emotional adjustment problems.

A few studies that examine the social relationships of adolescence and young adults with spina bifida have found very high rates of social isolation among individuals in this population.[1,2,9] Many youth with spina bifida who have been interviewed report strong feelings of loneliness and have very little peer involvement outside the school environment. Anderson and Spain[3] found that compared with matched control subjects, young adults with spina bifida were much less likely to have satisfying social relationships and were more dependent on family members for companionship. Many of the youth had never dated and felt they had no one to confide in regarding their social anxieties. More positive reports of quality of social life were found among youth who had less severe handicaps and attended regular schools vs. special schools.

The limited information presently available generally indicates that many young adults with spina bifida do not have a substantial number of meaningful interpersonal relationships. The most frequently reported problem among youth in this population is social isolation. This unavailability of satisfying peer relationships may cause additional stress to family members who may feel responsible for meeting the social needs of the person with spina bifida. Feelings of resentment may arise both on the part of the family who may feel burdened as well the individual with spina bifida who desires that these needs be met by peers.

D. External Support Systems
1. Educational Arena

For the child with spina bifida, experience in the educational arena will play an important role in determining long-term adjustment outcomes. Although the passage of Public Law 94-142 has brought increased attention and focus to the educational requirements of handicapped individuals, school systems continue to be challenged by the diverse needs presented by children with chronic illnesses such as spina bifida. Despite the fact that these individuals are now leading longer lives, many educational settings remain unprepared to offer them the experiences that are needed to make a successful transition from the high school environment to the social and economic realities of the adult world that lies beyond.

Although very little research has focused on aspects of the educational environment that enhance adjustment of young adults with spina bifida, a number of authors have outlined educational variables that may result in improved long-term functioning for these individuals. Physical access to buildings for children with mobility problems is one of the most basic of requirements in school settings. Also, teacher expectations and attitudes play a key role in determining student success, particularly for those who are handicapped.[2,18] If the teacher has knowledge of spina bifida and its implications, and adopts optimistic and realistic expectations of the child's academic ability, he or she will impact tremendously on the child's level of comfort in the school environment, self-esteem, and motivation.

The role of educational environments in assisting students in developing skills prerequisite for autonomy in adulthood becomes particularly critical when considering the long-term needs of youth with physical handicaps such as spina bifida.[3] Insofar as the child and adolescent receive individualized educational programs aimed at reinforcing academic strengths, increasing social confidence and independent living skills, identifying vocational interests and options for future work or education, and guidance with respect to relevant life issues such as parenting and sex, he or she will be more prepared to face the challenges of adulthood.

Many authors have also discussed the value of support services within the school for children with special needs.[3,19] Very few educational programs have counseling or social service programs that focus on the needs of handicapped individuals with conditions such as spina bifida. Psychosocial concerns of individuals and families are rarely included in individualized education programs, although functioning in these areas has a profound reciprocal relationship to academic motivation and success. Equally important is whether the health concerns of youth with spina bifida are addressed within the school setting. The degree to which school nursing staff are involved in supportive care activities such as dispensing medications, catheterization, monitoring of health status, and coordination with primary physicians and specialty care clinics influences the child and the family's perceptions of environmental support and is likely to positively impact on current and long-term adjustment.

Because of the interrelated needs of the child with spina bifida and the diverse services potentially available to address these needs, coordination of care becomes particularly salient. Very few educational environments have mechanisms for formally coordinating the academic program, therapies, support services, and medical needs of the child. In addition, rarely does monitoring of the individual progress of the child take place or follow-up once the child has left the high school environment. If educators adopt a future-oriented perspective regarding the needs of these children, their chances of success in adulthood are greatly increased.

There is some evidence to suggest that children with spina bifida who are enrolled in regular, integrated school environments where there are both physically handicapped and nonhandicapped students, function better academically, psychologically, and socially than their counterparts in special schools. Several studies have found that students with spina bifida in special school environments are much less likely to pass standardized tests than their counterparts in regular schools.[39] Anderson[1] found that a variety of problems were seen more frequently among children in boarding and special school settings than in regular school environments. Perhaps these findings are reflective of the severity of diagnoses found among handicapped students in special school environments rather than actual differences between these settings. However, Kinnealey and Morse[19] advanced the important point that if children with physical handicaps are to function in a heterogenous society, then their educational experience must include contact with the diverse populations that will be encountered in the real world.

2. Community Resources

The availability and utilization of community support resources is a factor likely to be influential in the long-term adjustment of children with spina bifida.[11] Community counseling programs, social service agencies, and community support organizations such as a spina bifida association are valuable support resources that can be of great assistance to children and families throughout the life span.

The types of community support services needed most consistently by young adults with spina bifida include medical, financial, educational, vocational, and mental health services. Unfortunately, there is a significant discrepancy between the needs presented by young adults with spina bifida and the preparedness of many community agencies to address these needs. Our present system of delivery in the U.S. is fragmented and limited in scope and the various services that are available for disabled patients during pediatric years become virtually nonexistent in adulthood. Many of the state funded multidisciplinary medical clinics for patients with spina bifida discontinue when the child reaches the legal age of adulthood; community counseling resources are limited and often lack professionals with expertise in working with children with physical handicaps; educational programs are often discontinued at age 18 except for those patients with high levels of cognitive functioning; and vocational resources often lack a comprehensiveness that would be of maximum benefit to the individual with spina bifida.

Despite the fact that many changes need to occur on a community level that would allow for greater support of handicapped adults, many communities are developing support programs that are addressing the needs of this population. Advocacy groups and organizations to address the comprehensive needs specific to people with spina bifida are influential in some states and have impacted on local legislatures. Unfortunately, many people with spina bifida reach adulthood unprepared to seek needed community support or to advocate for their own needs because of a lack of preparation and training in doing so. To the degree that comprehensive community service organizations become available, greater quality of life and psychosocial adjustment outcomes will be realized for adults with spina bifida.

In summary, there appear to be a number of potentially important factors that interact in a complex fashion and will influence the course of psychosocial adjustment for the child with spina bifida. As we have seen, healthy adult functioning for the individual with spina bifida is dependent on individual characteristics and competencies, family relationships, and social experiences, as well as the availability and utilization of adequate educational and community support resources. For the person with spina bifida, preparation for adulthood begins long before adolescence. The child is born with certain personality characteristics and temperament which, in part, determine self-perception of the world and shape interpersonal relationships. Experiences with family members and peers, in turn, mold the individual and are potential providers of support needed to buffer the stressful challenges of development. Experiences in the educational arena and utilization of available community resources also significantly impact on both the individual and his family. To maximize the possibility for more successful psychosocial outcomes and increase the quality of life for adults with spina bifida, focus should be given to all of the aforementioned areas throughout the course of the child's development.

III. CONCLUSIONS AND RECOMMENDATIONS

It is unrealistic to expect a young adult with spina bifida to live independently if they have not been prepared to do so throughout childhood. It is essential to address the needs that these children present in a number of different areas throughout their development in order to assist them in achieving more autonomous and satisfying lives as adults. It is the responsibility of parents and health care professionals to join forces and work together in such a way as to promote self-sufficiency on the part of the affected individual. Below we offer some suggestions with respect to meeting these needs (Table 1).

A. Medical

Multidisciplinary team intervention which includes such subspecialties as pediatrics, neurosurgery, orthopedics, urology, nutrition, physical therapy, psychology, and social work remains important in the medical management of the child throughout development. Health care professionals are encouraged to take an aggressive role in educating families and children about the varied aspects of spina bifida and provide them with reasonable explanations and rationale for medical procedures as well as aspects of psychosocial adjustment. It is also strongly recommended that health care providers work closely with parents to assist children in developing age-appropriate decision making skills in some areas of medical intervention and provide them with structured opportunities in the self-management of a variety of aspects of their disease (e.g., bowel and bladder, medication). Case management specialists become particularly important in the coordination of these services for families.

As the child with spina bifida approaches adolescence and adulthood, they present additional concerns that need to be addressed in the medical arena. Given the cognitive changes and new awarenesses that accompany development, the young adult often requires a re-education regarding the varied aspects of his disease. Health care professionals often assume that by the time the child with spina bifida reaches adolescence, he or she is very familiar with the many aspects of his or her medical condition and prognosis. However, teens often lack an adequate understanding of the disease and its implications. For the young adult of at least average cognitive ability, genetic counseling becomes critical. Equally important is education regarding the possibility of healthy sexual functioning and reproductive ability.

One of the most important needs of the young adult with spina bifida is continued medical care. It is essential that coordinated multidisciplinary team efforts be continued beyond pediatric years.

B. Emotional

Ideally, preventive intervention efforts targeted at known factors which place children at increased risk for emotional problems in adulthood would be of greatest benefit to children with spina bifida. Child focused groups aimed at enhancing social skills, self-esteem, and coping ability are helpful in increasing the person's perceptions of environmental control and would decrease the probability of the occurrence of some of the emotional and social problems that often accompany chronic illness. Some prevention intervention activity should

TABLE 1
Tasks for Psychosocial Intervention

Medical

1. Multidisciplinary team intervention beyond pediatric years
2. Education of families and children about spina bifida
3. Encouragement of medical compliance, age-appropriate decision making, and self-management behaviors
4. Case management
5. Genetic counseling
6. Education of young adults about prospects for sexual functioning and reproduction
7. Weight management programs

Emotional

1. Prevention programs for children and families (e.g., support/education groups)
2. Parent encouragement of self-help behaviors, daily living skills, and responsibility
3. Identification and appreciation of the child's individual strengths and abilities
4. Individual and family counseling
5. Peer support groups

Social

1. Development of social skills
2. Parent encouragement of involvement in social groups/organizations
3. Information regarding community resources
4. Adult day programs

Educational/Vocational

1. Psychological evaluation at regular intervals
2. Advocacy for appropriate educational programs and individualized educational programs
3. Programs aimed at increasing adaptive behaviors, social skills, and self-help ability
4. In-service workshops for school personnel/education of other students
5. Evaluation of vocational interests and abilities
6. Exposure to various work environments
7. Education regarding community resources
8. Coordination of services and follow-up beyond high school

also be focused on parents of children with spina bifida. Structured parent support/education groups might cover a broad range of topics common to parents of children with spina bifida including ways of developing self-esteem and self-help behaviors in children, successful methods of behavior management, and strategies of promoting compliance with daily routines (e.g., catheterization, medication). In addition, parents should receive early education and preparation for predictable stressful periods that lie ahead for themselves and their children. Groups designed to better prepare parents for these stressful periods (e.g., entering school, early adolescence, graduation from high school) might help to make these transitions much smoother and alleviate potentially negative emotional consequences.

Parents can impact significantly on their child's development of independence by teaching self-help and daily living skills and encouraging responsibility, age-appropriate decision making, and risk taking behavior. Furthermore, parents of children with spina bifida might create opportunities for their children to fully express their range of abilities and help them identify, appreciate, and capitalize on their personal strengths and talents. Most importantly, parents are encouraged to assist their children in developing a picture of their future from which they are able to begin setting goals.

Because of the overwhelming stresses and challenges that are frequently experienced by children with spina bifida and their families, individual and family counseling services are often required. Mental health professionals who are specially trained in working with children with chronic illness and their families should be an ongoing resource available throughout the life span. Many emerging adults would profit from individual counseling that addresses their feelings related to the social loss they have endured and social isolation they are experiencing. Many of these youths must receive help in coming to terms with their perceived discrepancy between the reality of their social world and the world which they often fantasize. Often unaddressed are the existential questions these youths have that center around the purpose and meaning of their lives as well as concerns about their own mortality. In addition to individual counseling, peer counseling by another individual with spina bifida would be beneficial in helping many youths address these feelings.

The emotional crisis experienced by many parents of young adults with spina bifida often goes unnoticed because of the extreme focus on the emerging adult. As a child reaches adulthood, many parents reexperience strong feelings related to the role the disease has played in their family. Emotions similar to that seen during the period of their child's birth often resurface as the parent begins the process of reorganizing their imagined picture of their child as an adult. Questions frequently arise concerning parental effectiveness and the level of involvement parents should now have in the young adult's life. If the child is dependent, many parents experience the additional anguish of worrying about who will care for their child in the future. Parents often require a great amount of reassurance, support, and counseling during this period.

C. Social

As is true for most people, the person with spina bifida has needs for social acceptance, companionship, and a sense of belonging. Families, mental health professionals, and communities should coordinate efforts in helping the child and young adult with spina bifida become more socially integrated. Parents must insure that their children are involved in social groups and organizations that offer opportunities for social interaction and the establishment of friendships. Mental health professionals are encouraged to work with parents to improve their child's level of social skill to ensure greater probabilities that they will be able to establish and maintain adequate social relationships.

It will be particularly important to provide some guidance to the young adult with regard to accessing community resources. Helping them become more aware of social activities available in the community and finding ways of motivating them to participate in these programs is particularly important. Barriers to participation in social and community activities include poor physical access and lack of transportation. Parents and professionals must join forces and advocate for better physical access to local facilities. For those young adults who are unable to drive, some instruction should be given in how to access community transportation systems.

Many young adults with spina bifida can profit from involvement in a long-term support group consisting of a peer network. In addition, counseling efforts focusing on issues such as dating, intimacy, body image, and sexual and marital adjustment are relevant for many of these young adults.

For some individuals with spina bifida, adult day programs or group home settings will provide the only opportunity for social interaction outside the home. More innovative programs need to be developed that specifically address the social needs of the young adult with spina bifida.

D. Educational/Vocational

Given the range of cognitive and academic ability found among children with spina bifida, it will be important that they receive psychological evaluation at regular intervals within the school setting. In addition to advocating for appropriate educational programs, parents should encourage school personnel to adopt individualized educational goals for these children. In addition to academic goals, these individualized educational programs should include activities aimed at helping the child develop adequate adaptive behavior, social skills, and self-help ability. Many of these children may also require additional support services within the school setting (e.g., counseling, social services).

Efforts should also be focused on training school personnel about chronic illness conditions such as spina bifida and its implications. In-service training workshops are helpful in this regard. In addition to developing a greater understanding of the disease, teachers and others should become more sensitive to the broader needs presented by these children. Teachers should work with parents to identify the child's strengths so that potential vocational interests might be identified at an early age. Educating other students about spina bifida is also important within the school setting.

Schools should accept the responsibility for assisting the adolescent with spina bifida in the transition to adulthood. Many of these children have spent their school years in special education classes and are ill-prepared to continue regular higher education programs or obtain employment. Schools can better prepare the adolescent for adulthood by identifying vocational interests and abilities, exposing the youth to a variety of work environments, familiarizing the adolescent with community resources, and providing opportunities for actual work experience during high school. Once high school is completed, the adolescent can profit from adult education and/or more extensive job training experiences. Educational advocates who can assist with financial, transportation, and career counseling resources are also needed to help the young adult reach goals beyond high school. For those individuals who have lower cognitive functioning, there needs to be a comprehensive focus on the development of adaptive behavior and daily living skills. Preparing these individuals for the possibility of unemployment and providing them with reasonable alternatives is particularly important.

In spite of the preparation for adulthood that is given to children with spina bifida by parents and professionals, a portion of these affected individuals never are capable of living autonomously. Subsequently, their overall care must be provided by family members or staff in a residential or institutional setting.

Three crucial questions often arise for families while caring for a chronically ill or handicapped adult family member: (1) is someone available to help with the care of the young adult if we become overwhelmed? (2) can we receive financial assistance to compensate us for our expenses related to the care of the affected individual? and (3) will we ever enjoy time for ourselves away from the young adult? We believe the answer to all of these questions can and should be "yes".

Because of personal reasons and/or the unavailability of community resources, many families choose to continue caring for the young adult with spina bifida. Given the amount of time and responsibility that this care entails, it is strongly felt that families should receive assistance in the home to lessen their burden. Daily caregiving in the home is probably the most stressful aspect of having a family member with spina bifida. Frequently the primary caregiver becomes overwhelmed by responsibilities and often feels resentful toward the disabled individual. In order to help prevent families from experiencing this stress, health aides to provide physical care and parent support/education in the home might prove to be beneficial and cost efficient.

It is strongly suggested that individual states begin examining the possibility of providing guaranteed medical insurance for affected individuals and funds for their medical supplies and adaptive equipment. State monies to supplement costs for such items as customized vehicles to transport adults with spina bifida and housing modifications would also greatly benefit families. Finally, we think it is reasonable for the state or federal government to pay the family a monthly stipend, similar to that paid to foster parents, if the affected adult does not meet the eligibility guidelines for SSI or other public programs.

For families who require time away from the young adult, respite care or adult foster homes equipped to handle special needs individuals would provide that outlet. Day programs or sheltered workshops to provide the affected individual with daytime activities such as recreation would also allow the family time away from the handicapped family member. We think families should be allowed the opportunity to decide for themselves when and for how long they need these services, and be encouraged to use them as they would any other community resource.

For those families unable to care for the young adult with spina bifida in the home, we would suggest that they utilize available residential facilities and adult foster homes within the community. However, these families may require supportive counseling to reach such a decision. Families will typically feel better about an out-of-home placement if resources specific to the needs of persons with spina bifida are available.

REFERENCES

1. **Anderson, E.,** The psychological and social adjustment of adolescents with cerebral palsy or spina bifida and hydrocephalus, *Int. J. Rehabil. Res.,* 2, 145, 1979.
2. **Anderson, E. and Clark, L.,** *Disability in Adolescence,* Methuen Press, New York, 1982.
3. **Anderson, E. M. and Spain, B.,** *The Child with Spina Bifida,* Methuen, London, 1977.
4. **Billings, A. G. and Moos, R. H.,** Psychosocial theory and research on depression: an integrative framework and review, *Clin. Psychol. Rev.,* 2, 213, 1982.
5. **Blum, R. W.,** The adolescent with spina bifida, *Clin. Pediatr.,* 22, 5, 1983.
6. **Breslau, N. and Marshall, I. A.,** Psychological disturbance in children with physical disabilities: continuity and change in a 5-year followup, *J. Abnorm. Child Psychol.,* 13, 199, 1985.
7. **Castree, B. J. and Walker, J. H.,** The young adult with spina bifida, *Br. Med. J.,* 283, 1040, 1981.
8. **Coleman, J. C.,** *The Nature of Adolescence,* Methuen, London, 1980.
9. **Dorner, S.,** Adolescents with spina bifida. How they see their situation, *Arch. Dis. Child.,* 51, 439, 1976.
10. **Dorner, S.,** The relationships of physical handicap to stress in families with an adolescent with spina bifida, *Dev. Med. Child Neurol.,* 17, 765, 1975.
11. **Drotar, D. and Bush, M.,** Issues in the care of children with chronic illness, in *Mental Health Issues and Services,* Hobbs, N. and Perrin, J. M., Eds., Jossey-Bass, San Francisco, 1985, 514.
12. **Drotar, D. and Crawford, P.,** Psychological adaptation of siblings of chronically ill children: research and practice implications, *Dev. Behav. Pediatr.,* 6, 355, 1985.
13. **Erikson, E.,** *Dimensions of a New Identity,* Norton, New York, 1974.
14. **Gayton, W.,** Management problems of mentally retarded children and their families, *Symp. Behav. Pediatr.,* 22, 561, 1975.
15. **Holroyd, J.,** The questionnaire on resources and stress: an instrument to measure family response to a handicapped family member, *Am. J. Community Psychol.,* 2, 92, 1974.
16. **Kazak, A. E.,** Families with disabled children: stress and social networks in three samples, *J. Abnorm. Child Psychol.,* 15, 137, 1987.
17. **Kazak, A. E. and Clark, M. W.,** Stress in families of children with myelomeningocele, *Dev. Med. Child Neurol.,* 28, 220, 1986.
18. **Kazak, A. E. and Marvin, R.,** Differences, difficulties, and adaptation: stress and social networks in families with a handicapped child, *Fam. Relat.,* 33, 67, 1984.

19. **Kinnealey, M. and Morse, A. B.,** Educational mainstreaming of physically handicapped children, *Am. J. Occup. Ther.,* 33, 6, June, 1979.
20. **Knowlton, D. D., Peterson, K., and Putbrese, A.,** Team management of cognitive dysfunction in children with spina bifida, *Rehab. Lit.,* 46, 259, 1985.
21. **Kolin, I. S., Scherzer, A., New, B., and Garfield, M.,** Studies of the school-age child with meningomyelocele social and emotional adaptation, *J. Pediatr.,* 78, 1013, 1971.
22. **Lax, R.,** Some aspects of the interaction between mother and impaired child: mother's narcissistic trauma, *Int. J. Psychoanal.,* 53, 339, 1972.
23. **Leftcourt, H. M.,** *Locus of Control: Current Trends in Theory and Research,* Lawrence Erlbaum, Hillsdale, NJ, 1976.
24. **MacBriar, B. R.,** *Issues in Comprehensive Pediatric Nursing,* Vol. 6, Hemisphere Publishing, New York, 1983, 1.
25. **Masters, J. C., Cerreto, M. C., and Mendlowitz, D. R.,** The role of the family in coping with childhood chronic illness, in *Coping with Chronic Disease: Research and Applications,* Burish, T. G. and Bradley, L. A., Eds., Academic Press, New York, 1983, 381.
26. **McAndrew, I.,** Children with a handicap and their families, *Child Care, Health Dev.,* 2, 213, 1976.
27. **McCormick, M. C., Charney, E. B., and Stemmler, M. M.,** Assessing the impact of a child with spina bifida on the family, *Dev. Med. Child Neurol.,* 28, 53, 1986.
28. **Meyerowitz, J. H. and Kaplan, H. B.,** Familial responses to stress: the case of cystic fibrosis, *Soc. Sci. Med.,* 1, 249, 1967.
29. **Myers, G. J. and Millsap, M.,** Spina bifida, in *Issues in the Care of Children with Chronic Illness,* Hobbs, N. and Perrin, J. M., Eds., Jossey-Bass, San Francisco, 1985, 214.
30. **Pearson, A., Carr, J., and Halliwell, M.,** The self concept of adolescents with spina bifida, *Z. Kinderchirurg.,* 40(Suppl. 1), 27, 1985.
31. **Pless, B.,** Clinical assessment: physical and psychological functioning, in *The Pediatric Clinics of North America Symposium on Chronic Disease in Children,* Haggerty, R. J., Ed., W. B. Saunders, Philadelphia, 1984.
32. **Pless, I. B. and Pinkerton, P.,** *Chronic Childhood Disorder — Promoting Patterns of Adjustment,* Henry Kimpton, London.
33. **Pless, I. B., Roghmann, K. J., and Haggerty, R. J.,** Chronic illness, family functioning and psychological adjustment: a model for the allocation of preventive mental health services, *Int. J. Epidemiol.,* 1, 271, 1972.
34. **Ramshorn, M. T.,** The individual in the family system, in *Psychiatric Nursing: Theory and Application,* Joel, L. A. and Collins, D. L., Eds., McGraw–Hill, New York, 1978, 243.
35. **Rosenberg, M.,** *Conceiving the Self,* Basic Books, New York,
36. **Seltzer, V.,** *Adolescent Social Development: Dynamic Functional Interaction,* Heath, Lexington, MA, 1982.
37. **Spaulding, B. R. and Morgan, S. B.,** Spina bifida children and their parents: a population prone to family dysfunction? *J. Pediatr. Psychol.,* 2(3), 359, 1986.
38. **Strax, T. E. and Wolfson, S. D.,** Life cycle crises of the disabled adolescent and young adult: implications for public policy, in *Chronic Illness and Disabilities in Childhood and Adolescence,* Blum, R., Ed., Grune & Stratton, Orlando, FL, 1984, 47.
39. **Tew, B.,** The adolescent with spina bifida: academic achievement, and employment prospects, *Br. J. Spec. Educ.,* 13, 22, 1986.
40. **Tew, B. and Laurence, K. M.,** Possible personality problems among 10-year-old spina bifida children, *Child Care, Health Dev.,* 11, 375, 1985.
41. **Tew, B. and Laurence, K. M.,** The relationship between intelligence and academic achievements in spina bifida adolescents, *Z. Kinderchirurg.,* 39(Suppl. 2), 122, 1984.
42. **Tew, B. J. and Laurence, K. M.,** The effects of hydrocephalus on intelligence, visual perception, and school attainment, *Dev. Med. Child Neurol.,* Suppl. 3, 129, 1975.

43. **Tew, B. J. and Laurence, K. M.,** Mothers, brothers and sisters of patients with spina bifida, *Dev. Med. Child Neurol.,* Suppl. 29, 69, 1973.
44. **Turk, J.,** Impact of cystic fibrosis on family functioning, *Pediatrics,* 34, 67, 1967.

INDEX